ARY

WE.600

COLOUR ATLAS OF
Surgical Exposures of the Limbs

COLOUR ATLAS OF
Surgical Exposures of the Limbs

Neil Rushton
MD, FRCS

Director of the Orthopaedic Research Unit
Fellow of Magdalene College
University of Cambridge
Honorary Consultant Orthopaedic Surgeon
Addenbrooke's Hospital
Cambridge, UK

Robert A. Greatorex
MA, FRCS

Senior Registrar in General Surgery
Addenbrooke's Hospital
Cambridge, UK

Nigel S. Broughton
FRCS

Senior Orthopaedic Registrar
Addenbrooke's Hospital
Cambridge, UK

Foreword by:
T. J. Fairbank
FRCS

Honorary Consultant Orthopaedic Surgeon
United Cambridge Hospitals and
 East Anglian Regional Board
Cambridge, UK

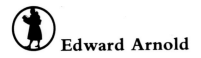
Edward Arnold

Gower Medical Publishing · London · New York

Distributed in all countries except USA, Canada and Japan by:
Edward Arnold (Publishers) Ltd.
41 Bedford Square
London WC1B 3DQ

Distributed in the USA and Canada by:
University Park Press
300 North Charles Street
Baltimore, Maryland 21201, USA

ISBN: 0-906923-20-4 (Gower)
0-7131-4440-8 (Edward Arnold)

British Library Cataloguing in Publication Data:

Rushton, Neil
    Colour atlas of surgical exposures of the limbs.
    1. Extremities (Anatomy)——Surgery——Atlases
    I. Title   II. Greatorex, Robert A.
    III. Broughton, Nigel S.
    617′.58059′0222   RD551

© Copyright 1985 by Gower Medical Publishing Limited.
34-42 Cleveland Street, London W1P 5FB, UK.
All rights reserved. No part of this publication may be reproduced,
stored in a retrieval system or transmitted in any form or by
any means electronic, mechanical, photocopying, recording or
otherwise, without the prior written permission of the publisher.

Printed in Hong Kong by Imago Publishing Ltd.

Project Editor: Sharyn Wong

Design: Leslie D. Watts

Illustration: Chris Furey
Lynda Payne

Foreword

The dissections and photographs presented in this book are of the highest class – indeed so good that the accompanying diagrams are scarcely necessary. The deliberately brief comments are practical and to the point. The authors are all young surgeons who learnt their surgical technique in recent years and remember what they found difficult or needed help over; they hand on that help here.

There are too many new medical books being pressed on the potential reader, who feels he must keep up-to-date, yet too often ends up in doubt as to whether he has got value for his money. I am happy to commend this book as a 'good buy' for anyone entering upon a surgical career, and any surgical department accepting trainees should surely have it available on their library shelves. There should be a copy, too, in the theatre for the theatre staff and perhaps another in the surgeon's room so that the embryo surgeon does not suffer the embarrassment of having to borrow it from Sister's office.

I have but one note of criticism. The authors apologise for sometimes extending the dissection illustrated unnecessarily far; they should not do so. The secret of safe surgery is adequate exposure, and a possibly unduly long scar should almost never be the source of criticism of the surgeon – on the contrary.

T. J. Fairbank
Cambridge

Preface

This book is intended for surgeons in training, medical students and all theatre staff, whatever their discipline. Our aim is to demonstrate regularly used surgical incisions using colour illustrations of cadaveric dissections together with a corresponding line diagram and a minimum of text. The choice of incisions included in this book was very difficult and we apologise for omitting the reader's favourite incision if this is the case. The dissections were performed on fresh cadavers in order that the natural colour should add realism to the dissection, the absence of blood allowing the relevant structures to be identified and giving a field which closely resembles that experienced when operating under tourniquet. A specially designed photographic system was used to produce illustrations of suitable quality.

This volume contains a basic set of approaches useful to most surgeons at some stage in their careers. Some incisions have been extended, beyond that which would normally be undertaken if treating a live patient, in order to demonstrate important anatomical points. These extra dissections have been clearly indicated in the text.

The choice of incision for any particular procedure must be left to the individual surgeon. It is not our intention to maintain that the illustrated incision is the best for every purpose, neither do we intend that this book should replace proper practical tuition; but it is our hope that it will supplement this time honoured and valuable teaching method. Textual comment has therefore been reduced to a minimum and we rely principally on the visual material to convey the steps in the performance of each incision.

Acknowledgements

We would like to acknowledge the cooperation and encouragement of the pathologists and their technicians at Addenbrooke's Hospital, Cambridge.

N.R., R.A.G. & N.S.B.
Cambridge, August, 1984

Contents

1 Exposures of the Upper Limb

1 Anterior Approach to the Shoulder Joint (Left)

Points to consider

- The coracoid is drilled before it is osteotomized so that an accurate reduction will result.

- Haemostasis should be maintained throughout the dissection.

Position

The patient is supine with a sandbag under the thoracic spine and the arm draped separately by the side.

1.2

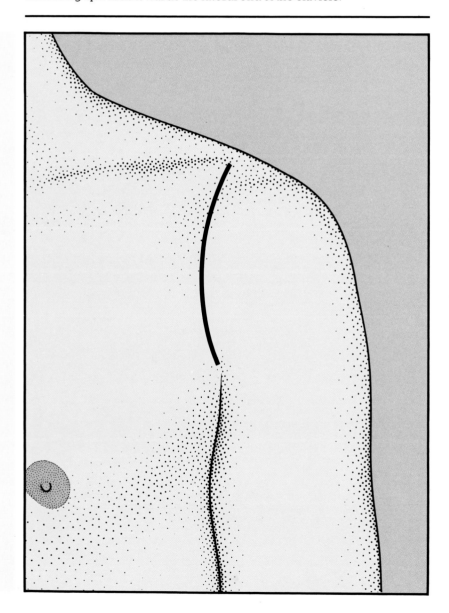

Fig. 1.2 Fat is cleared away to identify the cephalic vein in the deltopectoral groove.

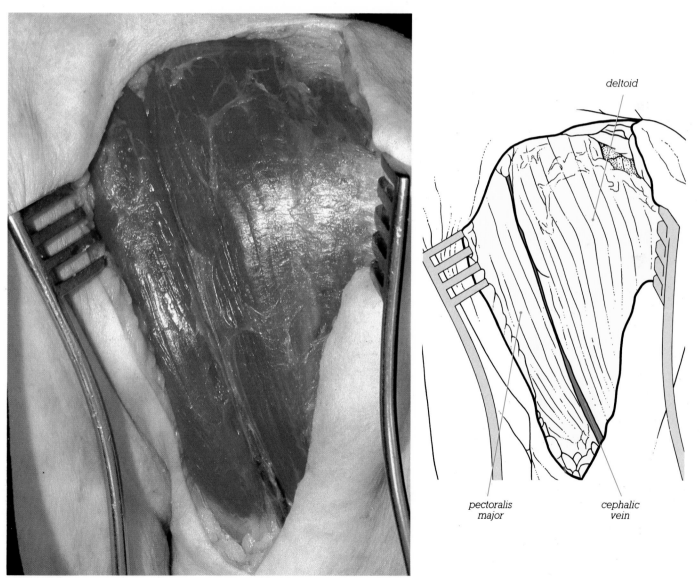

deltoid

pectoralis
major

cephalic
vein

Fig. 1.3 The deep fascia is incised 1 cm lateral to the cephalic vein. This strip and the underlying deltoid and cephalic vein are retracted medially and the bulk of deltoid retracted laterally. The coracoid process, with the origins of biceps and coracobrachialis, is identified. A hole is drilled into the coracoid process along its length of a size appropriate to the fixing screw to be used at the end of the dissection.

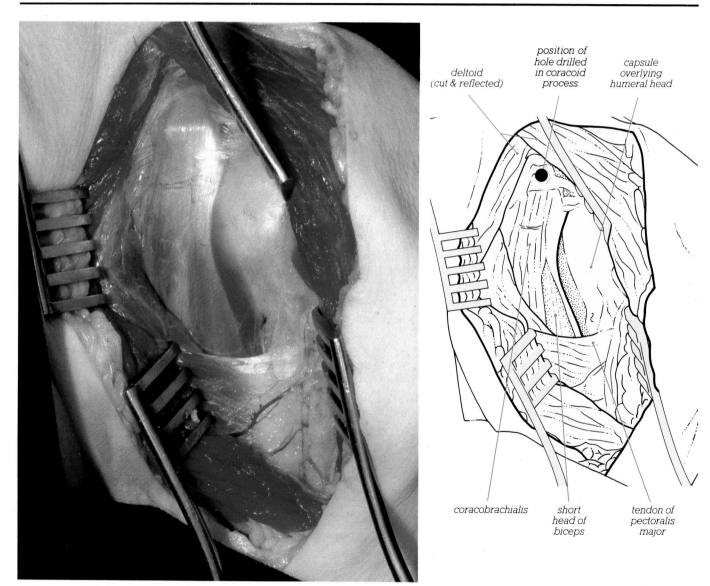

deltoid
(cut & reflected)

position of
hole drilled
in coracoid
process

capsule
overlying
humeral head

coracobrachialis

short
head of
biceps

tendon of
pectoralis
major

Fig. 1.4 The coracoid process is divided 1cm from its tip using an osteotome or oscillating saw. Biceps and coracobrachialis are reflected distally. Care must be taken to prevent accidental damage to the anterior circumflex artery.

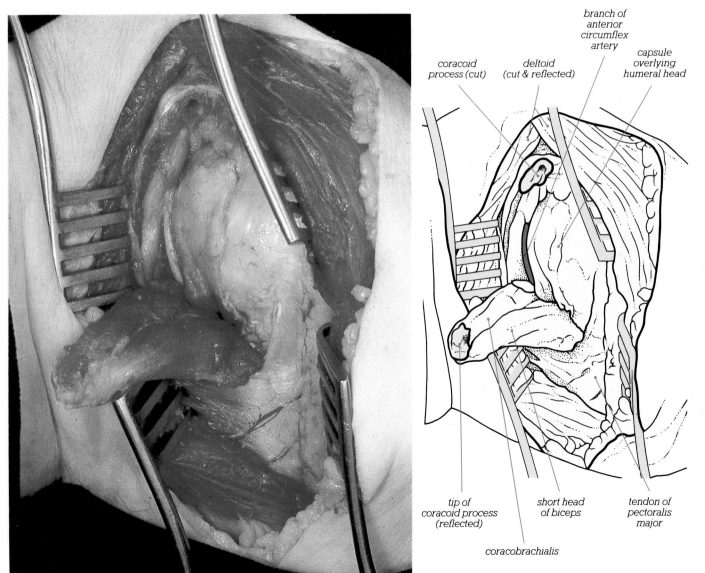

branch of anterior circumflex artery

capsule overlying humeral head

coracoid process (cut)

deltoid (cut & reflected)

tip of coracoid process (reflected)

short head of biceps

tendon of pectoralis major

coracobrachialis

Fig. 1.5 Subscapularis is divided 3mm from its insertion when the shoulder joint capsule is incised. External rotation of the humerus will expose the majority of the humeral head.

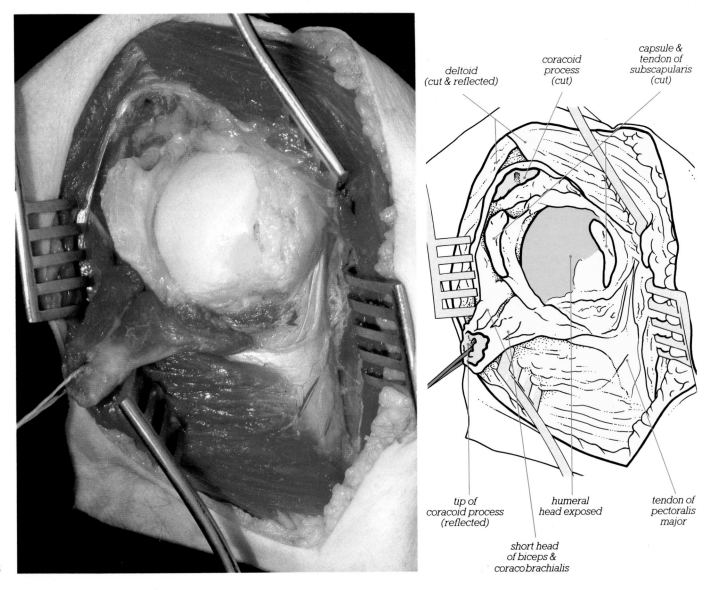

deltoid
(cut & reflected)

coracoid
process
(cut)

capsule &
tendon of
subscapularis
(cut)

tip of
coracoid process
(reflected)

humeral
head exposed

tendon of
pectoralis
major

short head
of biceps &
coracobrachialis

Fig. 1.6 The proximal shaft of the humerus can be displayed by incising through the insertion of pectoralis major, leaving 1 cm of its tendon attached to the humerus for later repair. A longitudinal incision down to the humerus will allow periosteal reflection.

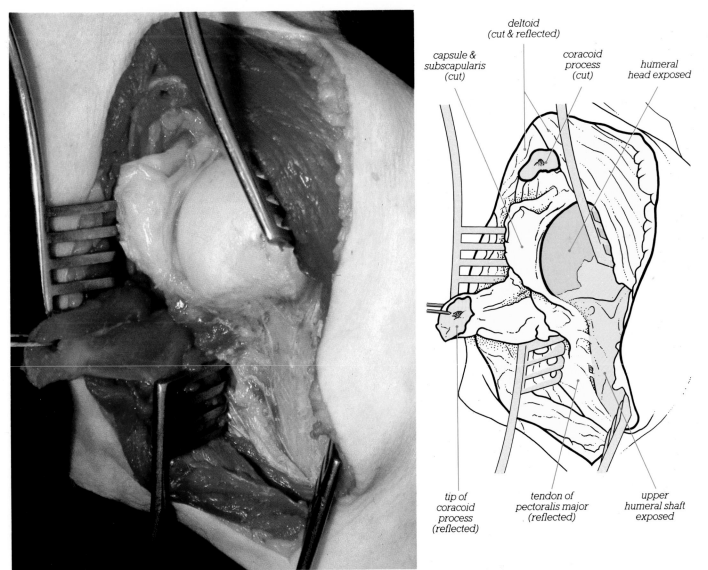

deltoid
(cut & reflected)

capsule &
subscapularis
(cut)

coracoid
process
(cut)

humeral
head exposed

tip of
coracoid
process
(reflected)

tendon of
pectoralis major
(reflected)

upper
humeral shaft
exposed

1.7

2 Posterior Approach to the Shoulder Joint (Left)

Fig. 2.1 The incision runs around the lateral margin of the acromion and along the spine of the scapula to the medial border.

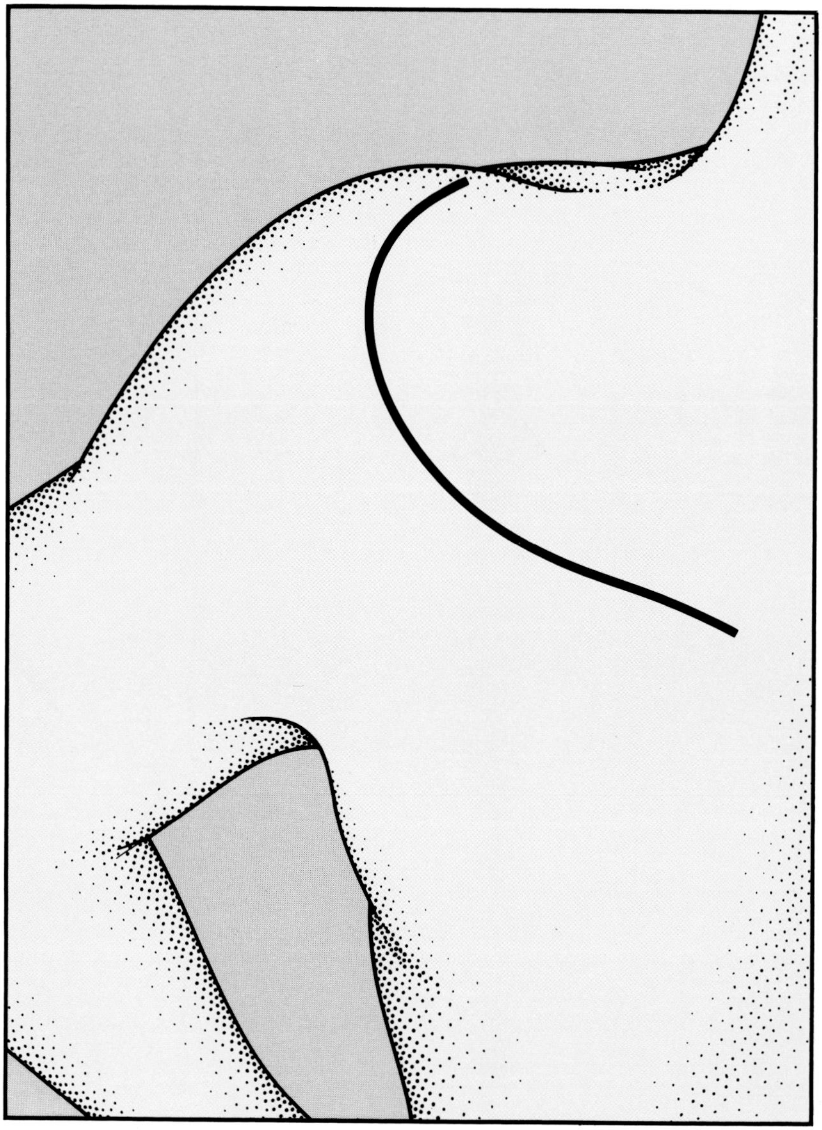

Points to consider

- The arm should be draped separately to allow manipulation during dissection as rotation will permit inspection of the majority of the humeral head.

- The incision is often done for posterior dislocation of the humeral head, which can then be felt in its dislocated position.

Position
The patient lies with the affected side uppermost and the arm draped separately by the side.

Fig. 2.2 Trapezius and deltoid are identified. Deltoid is detached subperiosteally from the scapula and is reflected distally.

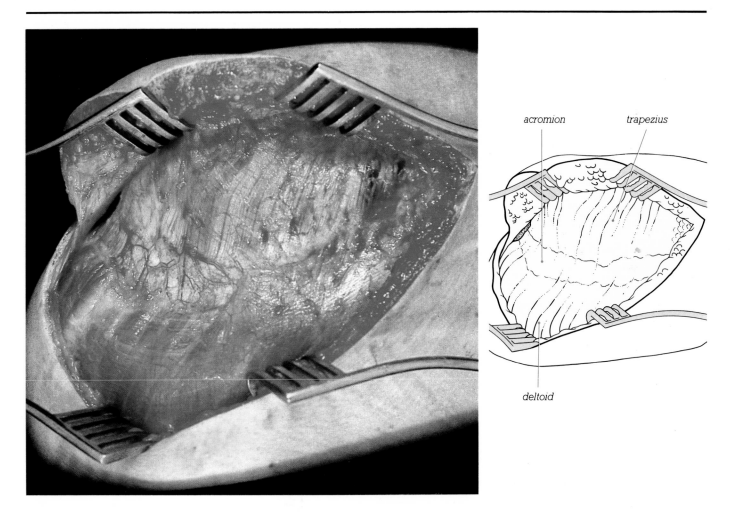

acromion   trapezius

deltoid

Fig. 2.3 Infraspinatus and its tendon are identified.

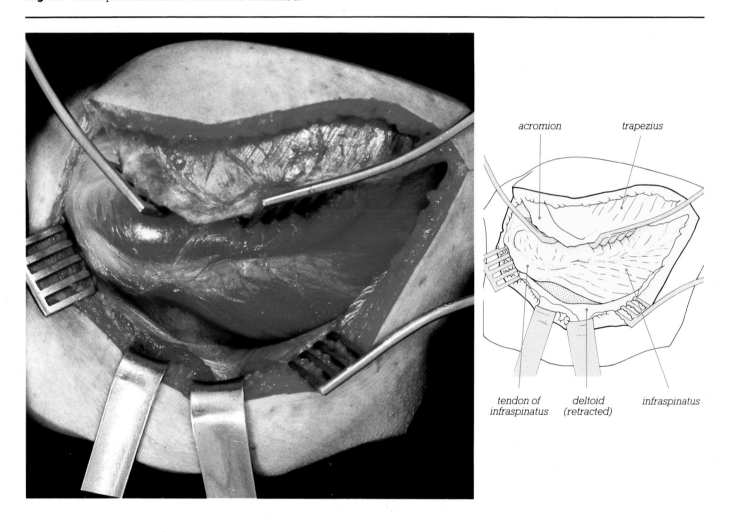

acromion

trapezius

tendon of
infraspinatus

deltoid
(retracted)

infraspinatus

Fig. 2.4 The infraspinatus tendon is divided at its insertion close to the greater tuberosity and retracted medially.

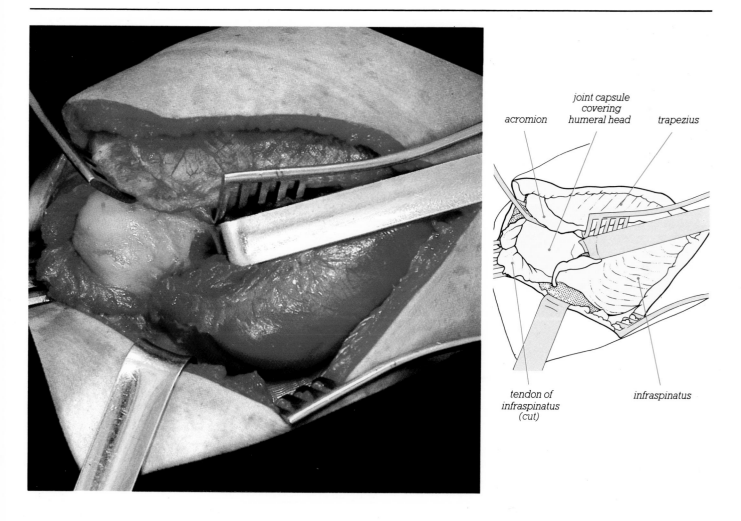

acromion

joint capsule
covering
humeral head

trapezius

tendon of
infraspinatus
(cut)

infraspinatus

Fig. 2.5 The joint capsule is incised. This incision can be enlarged and the humeral head exposed.

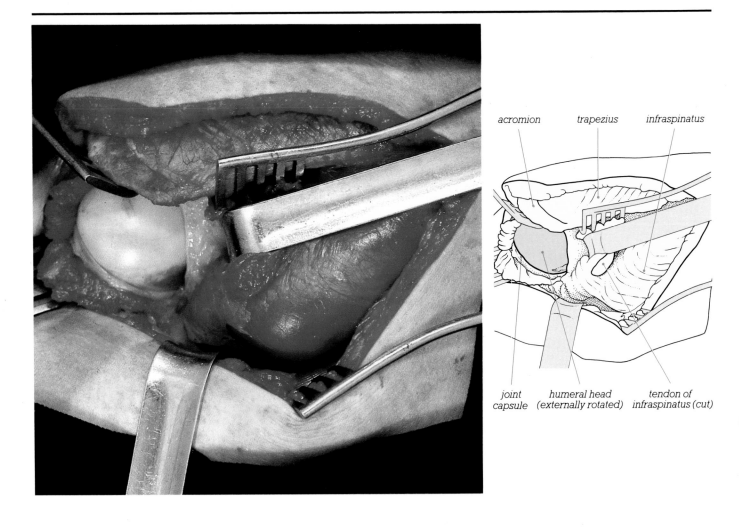

acromion   trapezius   infraspinatus

joint capsule   humeral head (externally rotated)   tendon of infraspinatus (cut)

3 Approach to the Subclavian Vessels (Right)

Fig. 3.1 The incision is 1cm above and parallel to the upper border of the medial two-thirds of the clavicle.

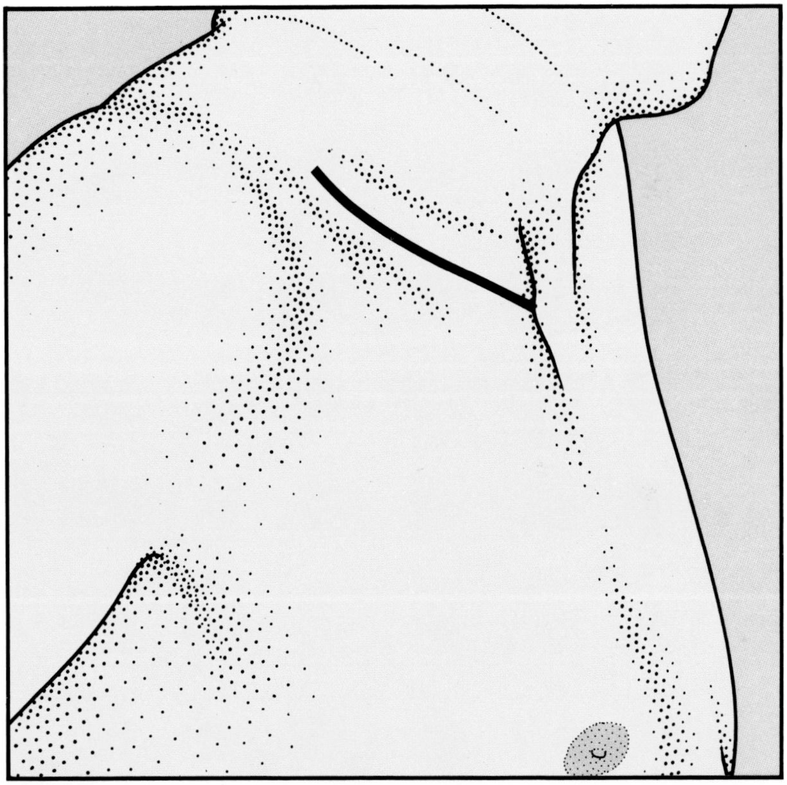

Points to consider

- The anatomy of the subclavian vessels is not identical on both sides (see Fig. 3.1a).

- Careful dissection and scrupulous haemostasis is required to prevent inadvertent damage to vulnerable and important neurovascular structures.

- Traction on the arm may be required to improve exposure of the deeper structures.

Position

The patient is supine with a sandbag between the shoulders, the face turned away and the neck extended slightly. The whole table is tilted so that the patient's feet point downwards.

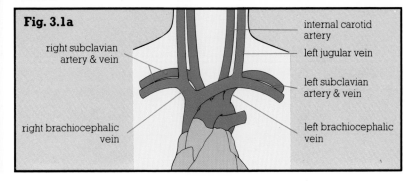

Fig. 3.1a

- internal carotid artery
- right subclavian artery & vein
- left jugular vein
- left subclavian artery & vein
- right brachiocephalic vein
- left brachiocephalic vein

Fig. 3.2 The skin and platysma are divided as are the superior clavicular nerves.

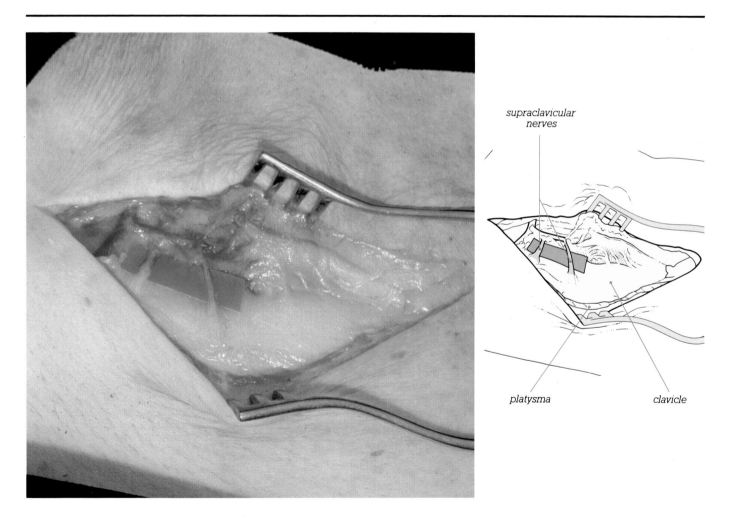

supraclavicular
nerves

platysma

clavicle

Fig. 3.3 If necessary, the external jugular vein is ligated and divided and the deep fascia incised. Omohyoid and the lateral edge of sternomastoid are identified and any transverse cervical vessels which impede access are ligated and divided.

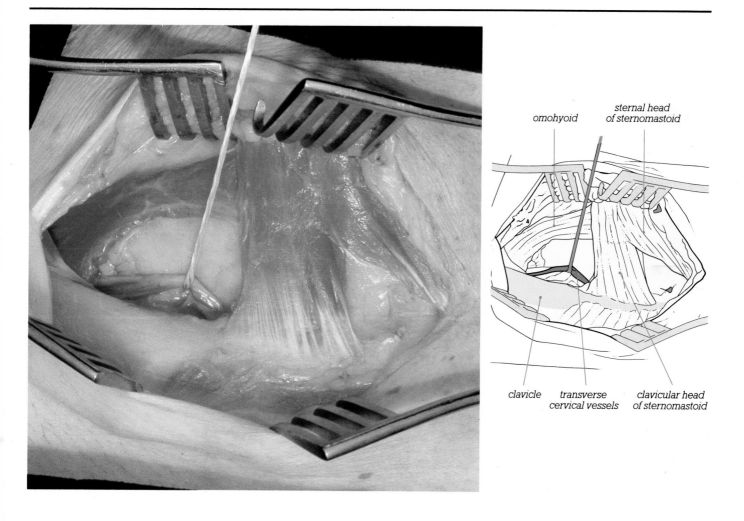

omohyoid

sternal head
of sternomastoid

clavicle

transverse
cervical vessels

clavicular head
of sternomastoid

Fig. 3.4 The clavicular attachment of sternomastoid is divided close to the bone and retracted to expose the internal jugular vein. Upward retraction of omohyoid will reveal the lower trunk of the brachial plexus.

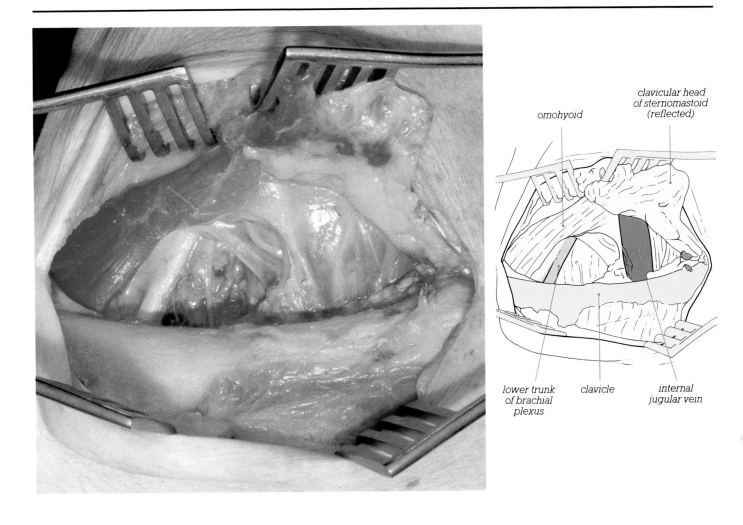

Fig. 3.5 Using a saw the clavicle is divided just lateral to its midpoint. The capsule of the sternoclavicular joint and the costoclavicular ligament are divided, and the medial portion of the clavicle removed by dividing the attachments of pectoralis major and subclavius. This will reveal a subclavian vein. Gentle retraction on the internal jugular vein will allow the phrenic nerve to be seen lying on scalenus anterior.

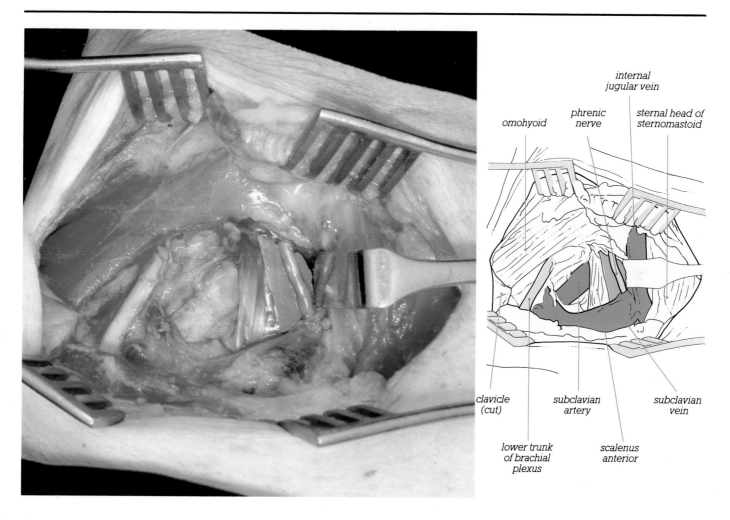

Fig. 3.6 Scalenus anterior is divided, taking care not to damage the phrenic nerve, allowing the second and third parts of the subclavian artery to be seen. Slings can be placed around the artery proximally and distally and around all its tributaries if an arteriotomy is to be performed.

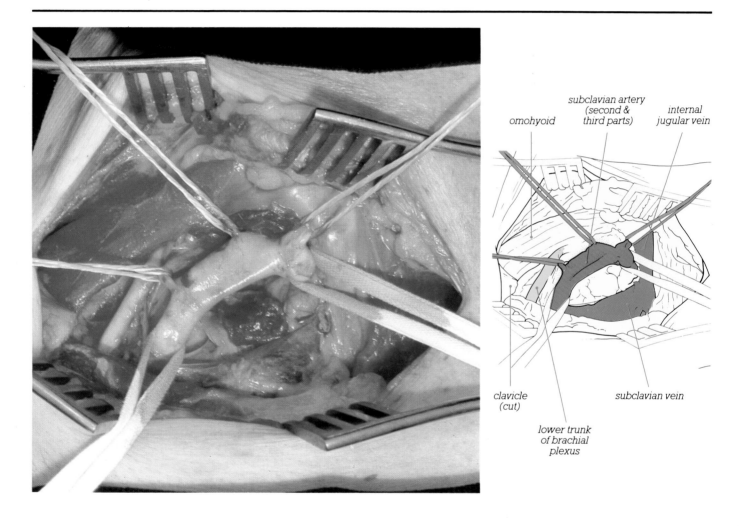

4 Exploration (Block Dissection) of the Axilla (Right)

Fig. 4.1 The 10cm incision is along the lateral border of pectoralis major and centred over the axilla.

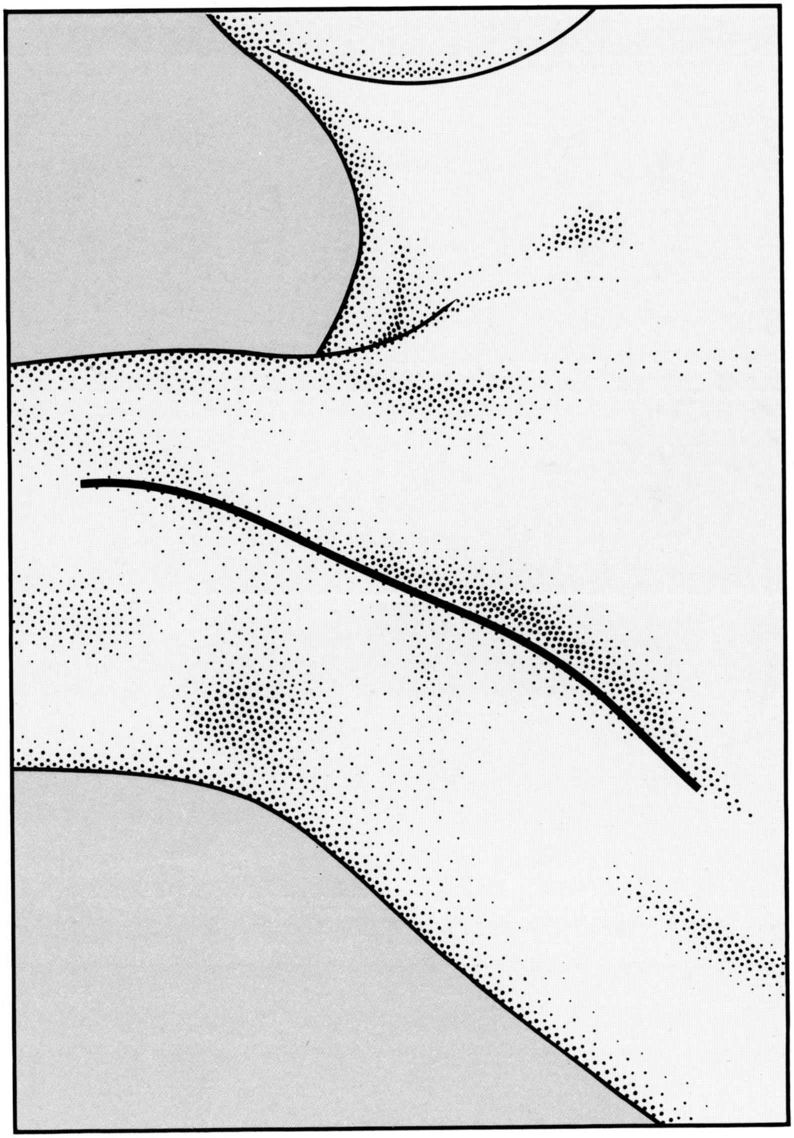

Points to consider

- Careful haemostasis is required to allow the best possible view of this complicated region.

- It is essential to identify structures before they are divided or damaged. It is particularly important that the major neurovascular structures not be damaged inadvertently.

Position
The patient is supine with the arm abducted to ninety degrees, fully externally rotated, on an arm board.

1.19

Fig. 4.2 The edge of pectoralis major is defined and the deep fascia incised to gain access to the axilla.

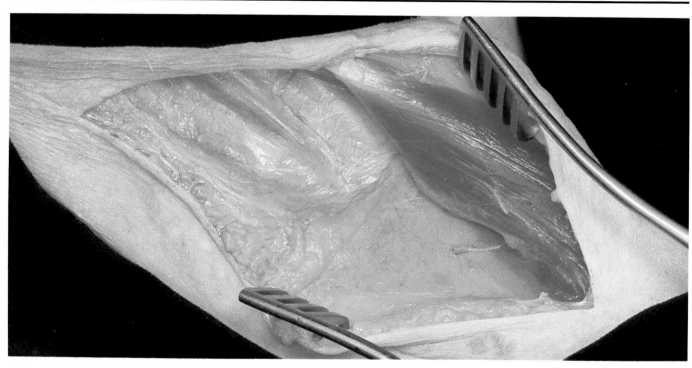

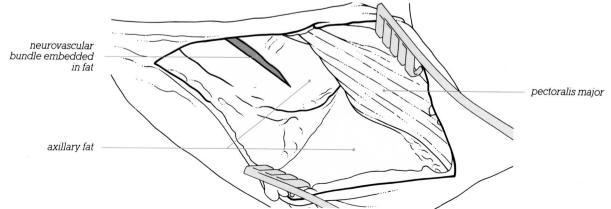

neurovascular bundle embedded in fat

axillary fat

pectoralis major

Fig. 4.3 Pectoralis major is elevated and pectoralis minor identified on the lateral thoracic wall. A subcutaneous dissection is made through the fat posteriorly before reaching latissimus dorsi, indicating the posterior limit of the axilla.

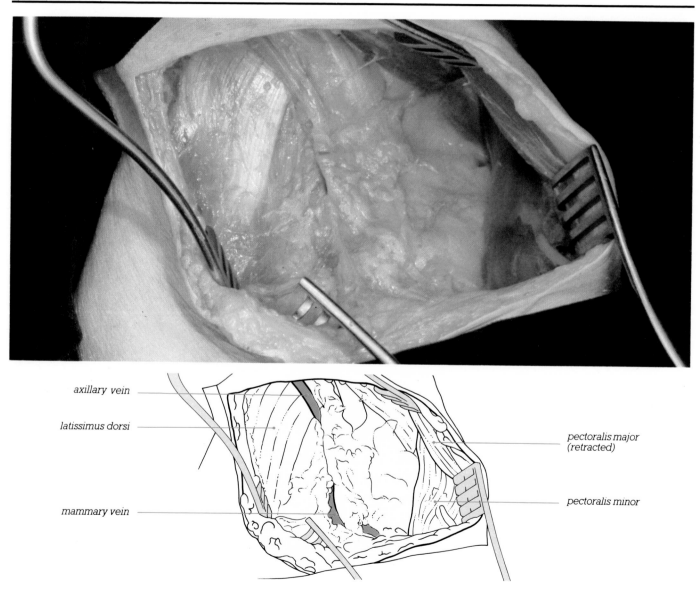

axillary vein

latissimus dorsi

mammary vein

pectoralis major (retracted)

pectoralis minor

1.21

Fig. 4.4 Pectoralis minor is followed to its attachment to the coracoid process from which it is detached. The neurovascular bundle can be seen and palpated.

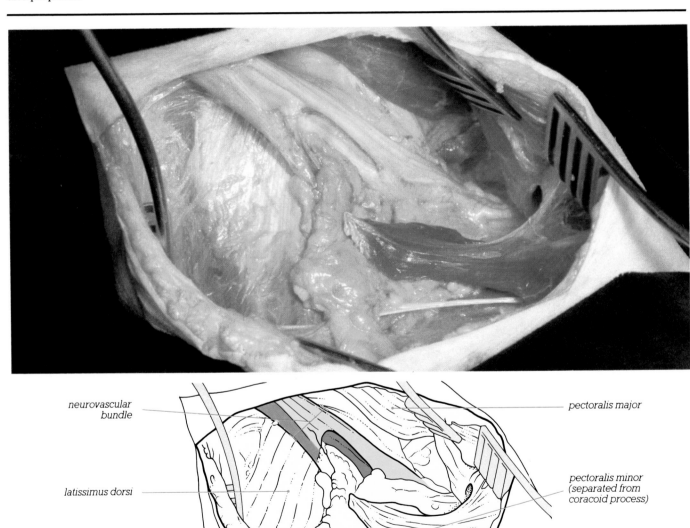

neurovascular bundle

pectoralis major

latissimus dorsi

pectoralis minor (separated from coracoid process)

intercostobrachial nerve

Fig. 4.5 Fatty tissue, including the lymph nodes, is cleared from the axillary vein, avoiding damage to the axillary artery and the cords of the brachial plexus. Axillary fat is cleared working downwards from the vein, small veins and arteries being ligated and divided in the process. Intercostobrachial nerves and lateral thoracic vessels must be divided, taking care to avoid damage to the long thoracic nerve and the nerves of latissimus dorsi. As the fat is cleared, latissimus dorsi, subscapularis and serratus anterior come into view.

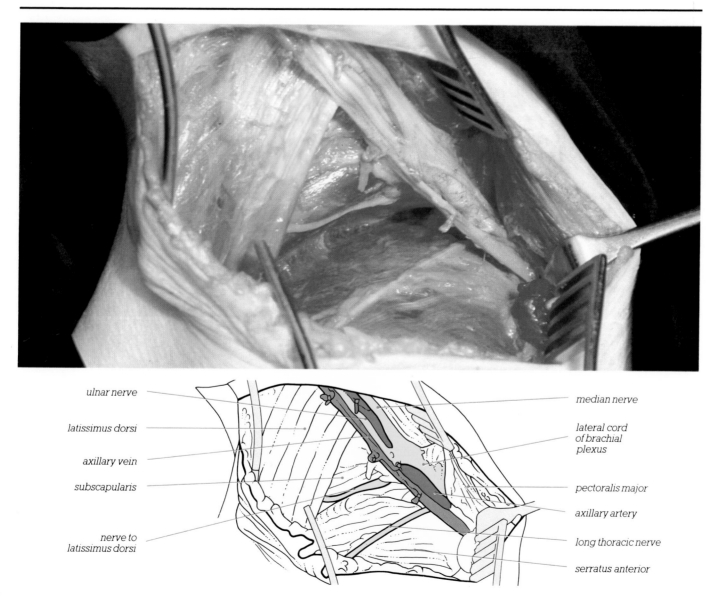

ulnar nerve

latissimus dorsi

axillary vein

subscapularis

nerve to latissimus dorsi

median nerve

lateral cord of brachial plexus

pectoralis major

axillary artery

long thoracic nerve

serratus anterior

5 Exposure of the Axillary Artery and Proximal Part of the Brachial Artery (Left)

Points to consider

- The artery is surrounded by the axillary vein and the median and ulnar nerves so great care must be taken when isolating the vessels.

- The arteriotomy is usually sutured with fine suture (for example, 5.0) and the wound closed with a suction drain.

Position
The patient is supine with the arm abducted to ninety degrees and externally rotated.

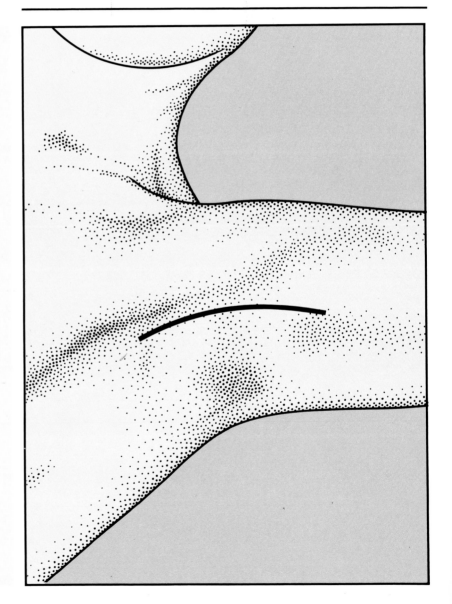

Fig. 5.1 The lateral border of pectoralis major is identified. The 10cm skin incision runs along the line of the brachial artery and lies close to the edge of pectoralis major, extending distally.

Fig. 5.2 Pectoralis major is retracted proximally and dissection continues down through the fat to the artery. Using the artery as a landmark it is freed from its surrounding veins and nerves. Slings are placed around the vessel proximally and distally and around any small branches. Should an arteriotomy be required, it is made transversely and will, for example, allow an embolectomy catheter to be inserted.

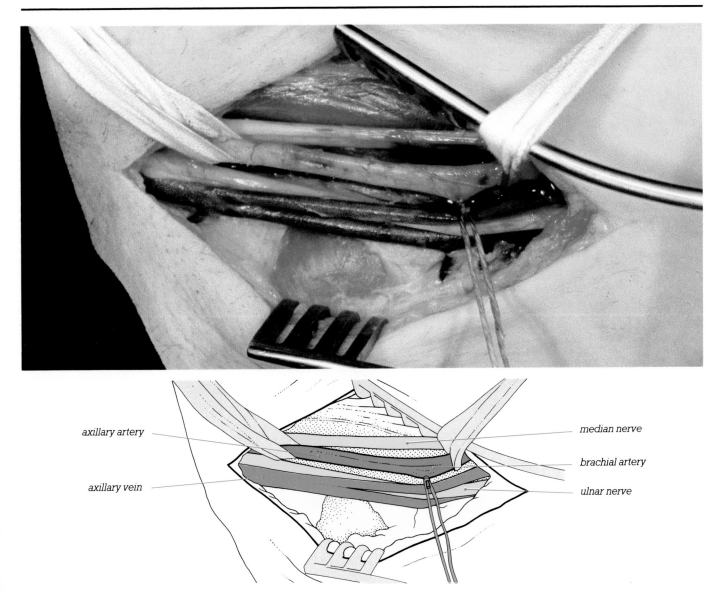

axillary artery

axillary vein

median nerve

brachial artery

ulnar nerve

1.25

6 Anterolateral Approach to the Humeral Shaft (Right)

Fig. 6.1 The incision is 1cm lateral to the palpated lateral edge of biceps, just proximal to the deltoid insertion and extending distally towards the antecubital fossa.

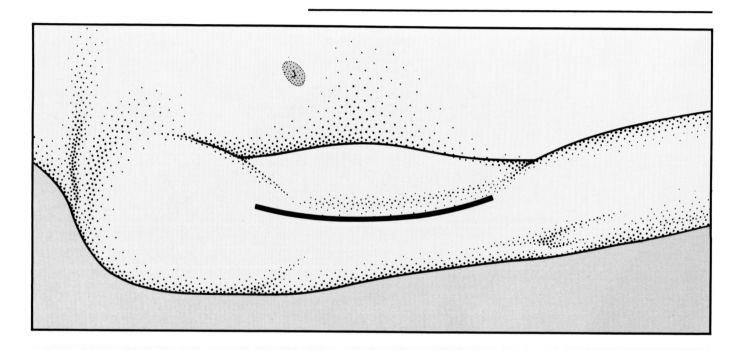

Points to consider

- The lateral cutaneous branch of the musculocutaneous nerve can be preserved if it is identified in the lower part of the wound.

- There is often a large vein in the upper part of brachialis which should be tied.

- If the elbow is flexed, access to the humerus is increased.

- As the radial nerve lies between brachialis and triceps, it is protected by the lateral part of the split brachialis.

- The incision may be extended proximally in the deltopectoral groove to give access to the upper humeral shaft.

Position

The patient is supine with the limb on an arm table. If only the lower part of the incision is required, a high tourniquet may be used.

Fig. 6.2 The deltoid insertion, biceps and brachialis are identified.

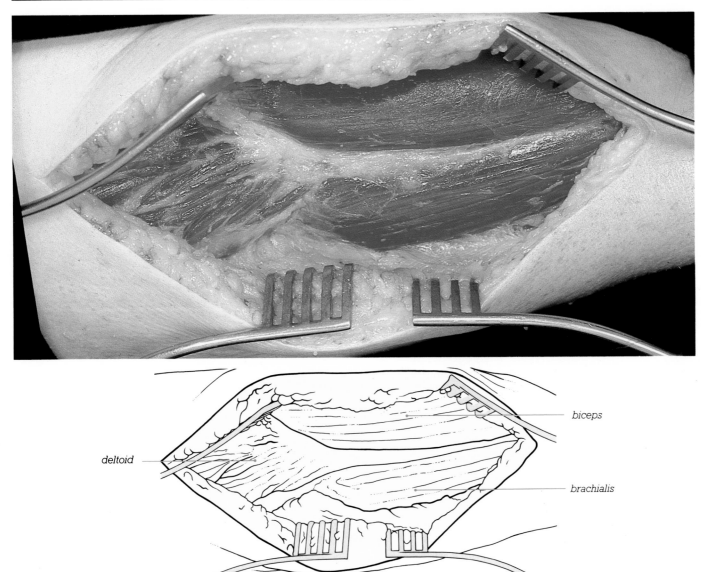

deltoid

biceps

brachialis

Fig. 6.3 Brachialis is split longitudinally in the line of its fibres from its anterolateral surface to the bone. This cleft in brachialis can be extended distally to within 4cm of the epicondyle without entering the elbow joint.

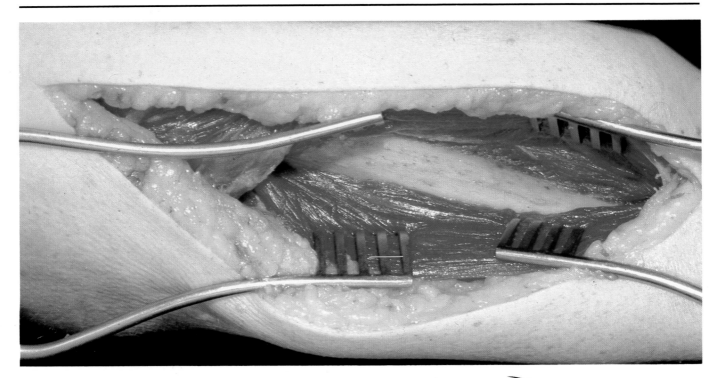

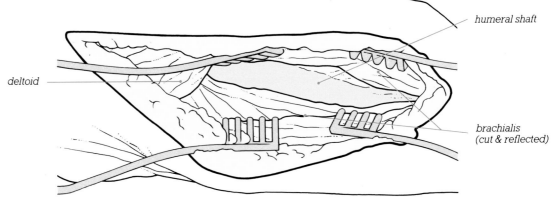

deltoid

humeral shaft

brachialis
(cut & reflected)

7 Posterior Approach to the Humeral Shaft (Right)

Fig. 7.1 Having identified the long head of triceps by its surface marking, the longitudinal incision is made in the posterior aspect of the arm along the lateral edge of the long head extending from the deltoid insertion to the olecranon.

Points to consider

- The radial nerve is vulnerable in the deep part of the dissection proximally and must be identified before proceeding.

- As long as the deep dissection remains in the midline there are no other important structures distally as far as the olecranon.

Position

The patient is prone with the arm abducted, the elbow flexed and supported over the edge of the table. A high tourniquet can be applied unless the most proximal part of the exposure is required.

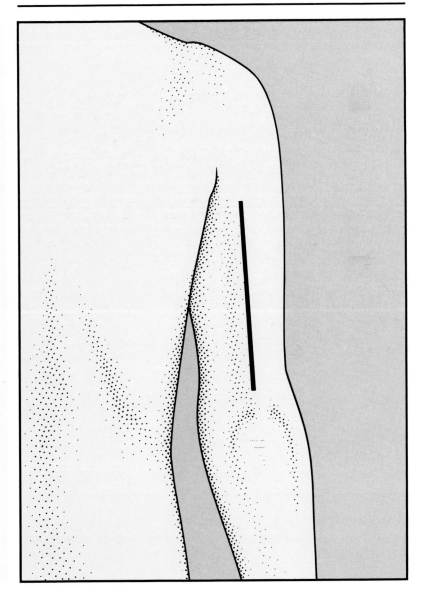

Fig. 7.2 The long and lateral heads of triceps are identified. A small incision is made through the deep fascia over the lateral edge of the proximal part of the long head. The fascia is split distally, taking care not to cut into the underlying soft tissue.

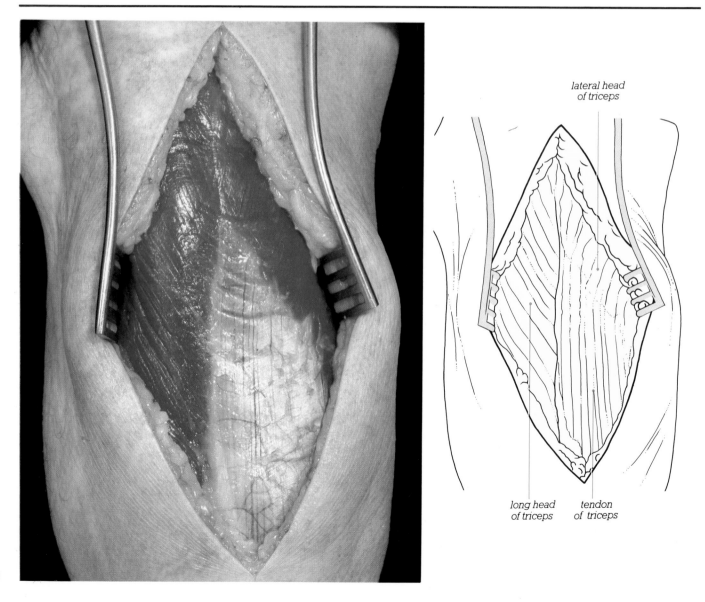

lateral head
of triceps

long head
of triceps

tendon
of triceps

Fig. 7.3 The long and lateral heads can now be separated to reveal the deep head of triceps at the upper end of the wound. Great care must be taken to avoid the neurovascular bundle, containing the radial nerve and profunda vessels, which runs obliquely from medial to lateral across the proximal part of the deep head.

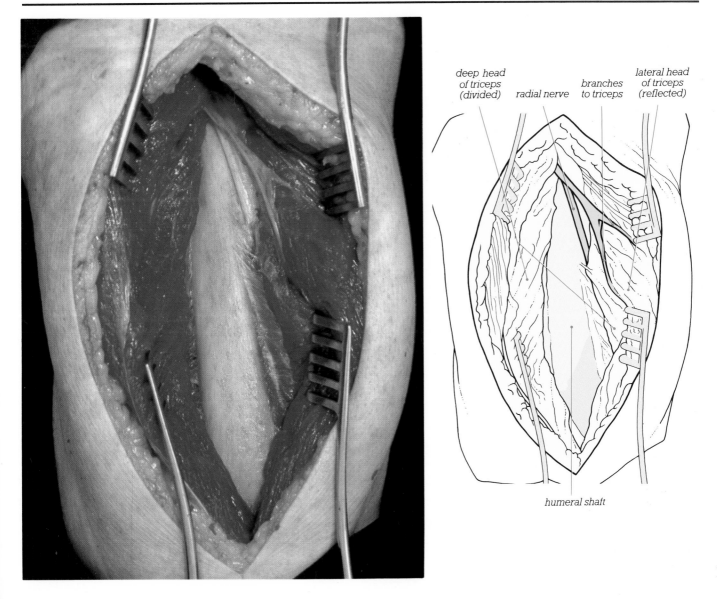

deep head
of triceps
(divided) radial nerve branches
to triceps lateral head
of triceps
(reflected)

humeral shaft

1.31

Fig. 7.4 The neurovascular bundle should be protected and an incision made in the midline through the deep head down to the bone. This incision can be continued distally to expose the shaft of the humerus as far as the olecranon.

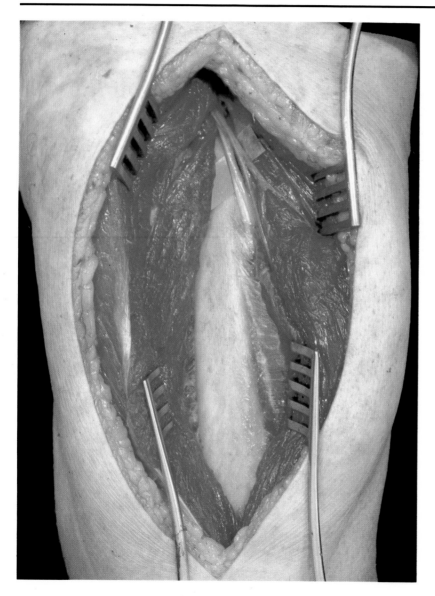

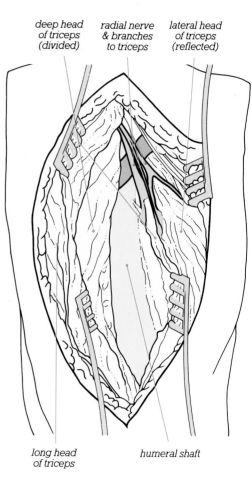

deep head of triceps (divided)

radial nerve & branches to triceps

lateral head of triceps (reflected)

long head of triceps

humeral shaft

8 Exposure of the Olecranon (Right)

Fig. 8.1 The incision is centred over the olecranon in the long axis of the arm.

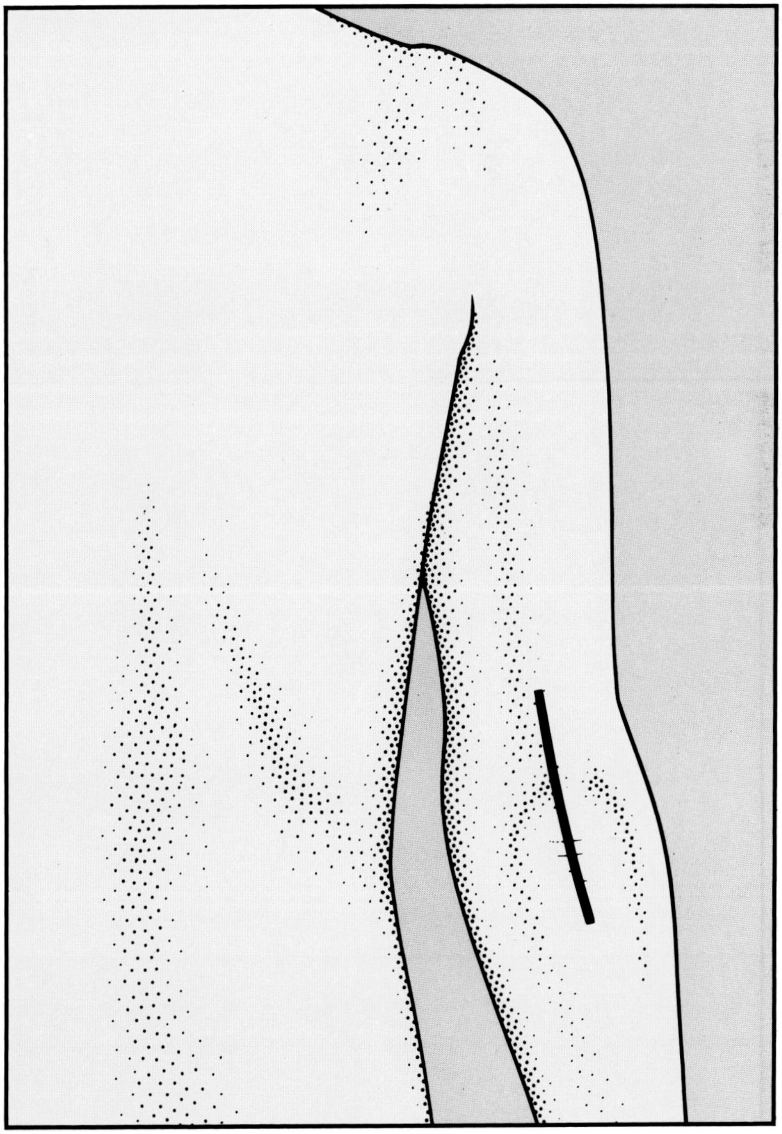

Points to consider

- If the dissection is to stray from the midline of the olecranon, the ulnar nerve should first be identified.

- Extension along the olecranon process can be carried along the full extent of the ulna (see Fig. 17.3).

Position
The patient is supine with the arm flexed over the chest and a tourniquet applied to the upper arm.

1.33

Fig. 8.2 The triceps tendon is identified with the fibres of the long head joining it medially.

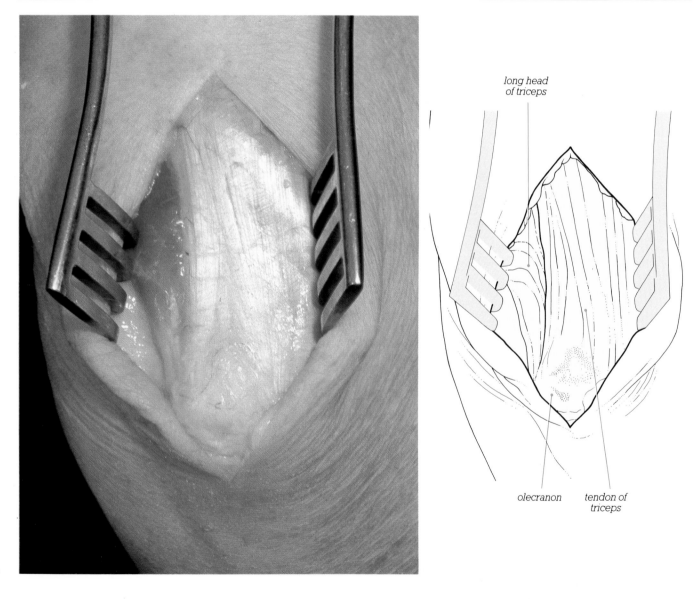

long head
of triceps

olecranon   tendon of
triceps

Fig. 8.3 The triceps tendon is incised in the long axis of the limb over the point of the olecranon process. A subperiosteal dissection will display the olecranon process.

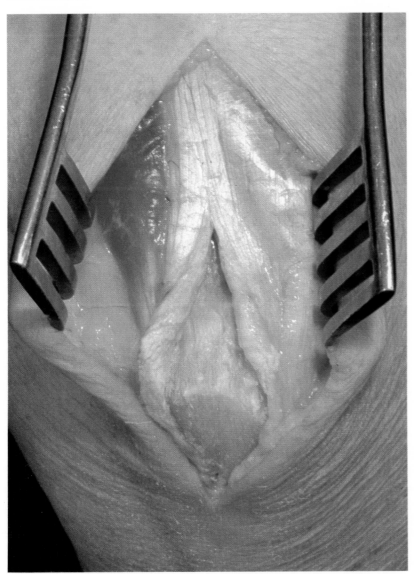

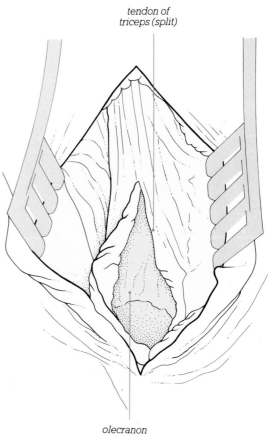

tendon of
triceps (split)

olecranon

Fig. 8.4 The ulnar nerve may be exposed deliberately, but care must be taken to avoid inadvertent damage to it.

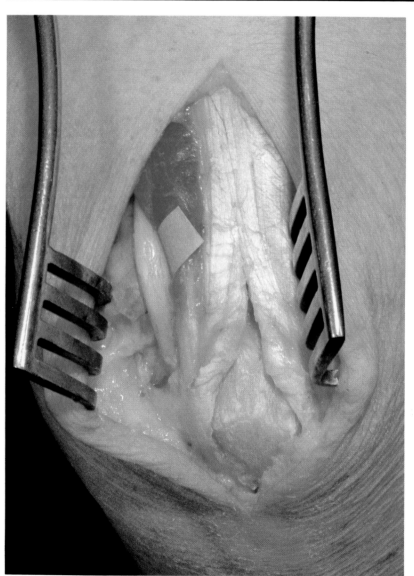

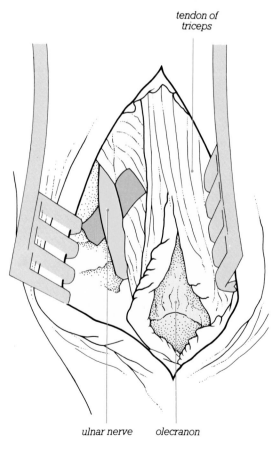

tendon of
triceps

ulnar nerve   olecranon

9 Approach to the Supracondylar Region of the Humerus and Posterior Aspect of the Elbow Joint (Left)

Points to consider

- Great care must be taken to preserve the ulnar nerve in the medial aspect of the dissection.

- The exposure may be extended proximally subperiosteally without further damage to triceps

Position
The patient is supine with the affected arm across the chest and a tourniquet applied.

Fig. 9.1 The 12cm incision starts at the point of the olecranon and extends proximally in the posterior line of the limb.

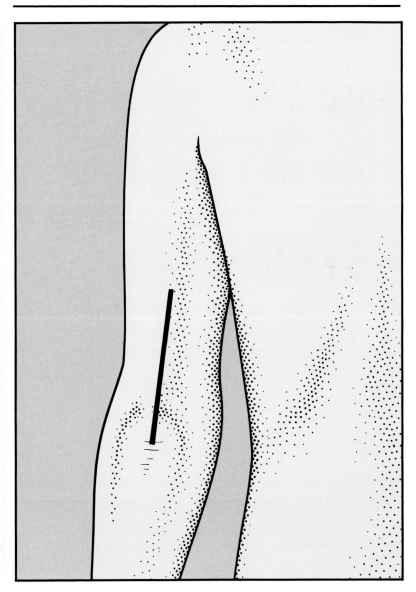

1.37

Fig. 9.2 The incision is deepened until the tendon of triceps and the olecranon are exposed.

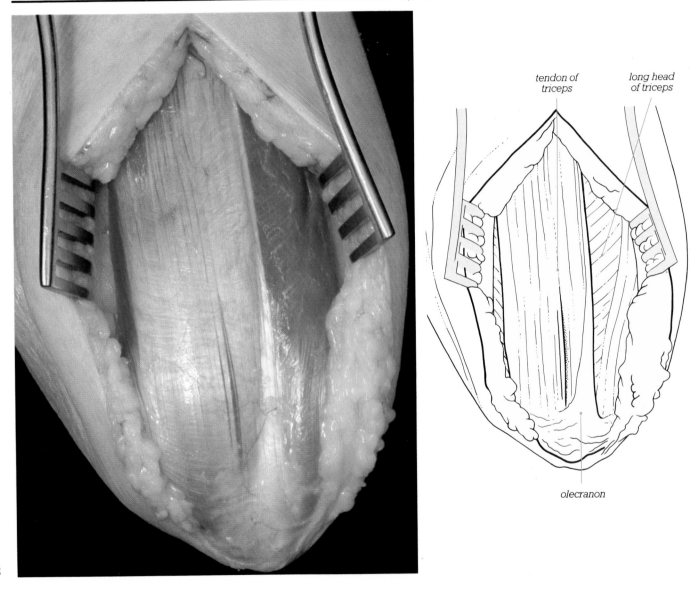

tendon of
triceps

long head
of triceps

olecranon

Fig. 9.3 A V-shaped incision is made in the distal part of the triceps tendon with the apex of the V proximal.

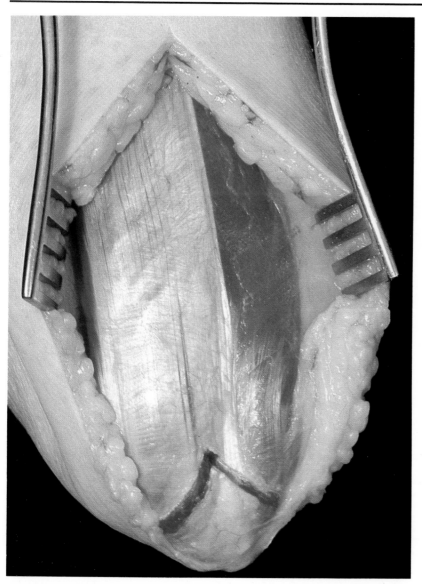

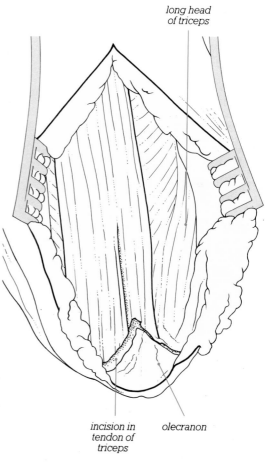

long head
of triceps

incision in
tendon of
triceps

olecranon

1.39

Fig. 9.4 The tendon is reflected. The periosteum is elevated, detaching
the medial head of triceps from the supracondylar part of the humerus. If
the elbow joint is to be exposed, the capsule is incised as triceps is
reflected; otherwise, the capsule is left intact.

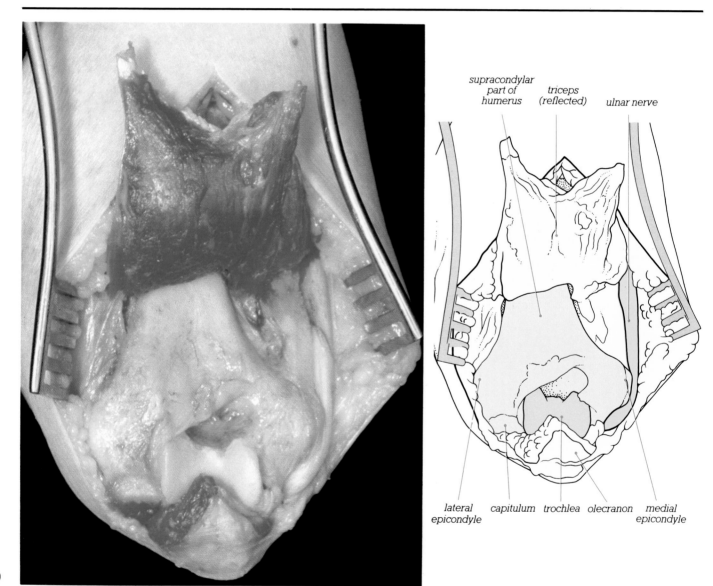

supracondylar
part of
humerus

triceps
(reflected)

ulnar nerve

lateral
epicondyle

capitulum trochlea olecranon

medial
epicondyle

Transolecranon Approach to the Elbow Joint (Right)

Points to consider

- Extensions and dissections medially should proceed with caution to avoid damage to the ulnar nerve.

- The hole is drilled before the olecranon is divided to allow accurate realignment of the articular surface.

- The size of the drill hole is governed by the size of the screw to be used to reattach the tip of the olecranon.

Position
The patient lies with the arm across the chest, elbow flexed to ninety degrees, and a tourniquet applied.

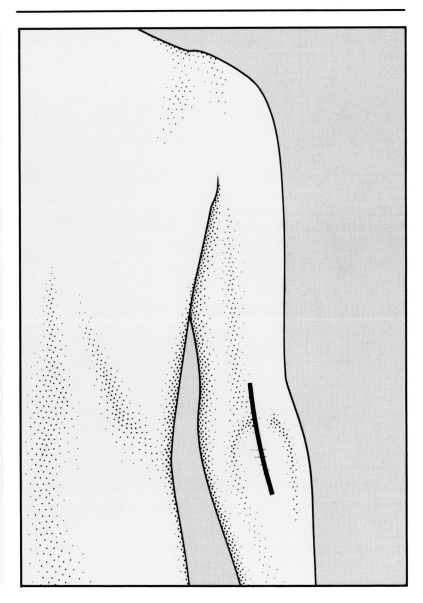

Fig. 10.1 The 10cm incision is centred over the olecranon in the long axis of the limb.

Fig. 10.2 The olecranon and triceps tendon are identified.

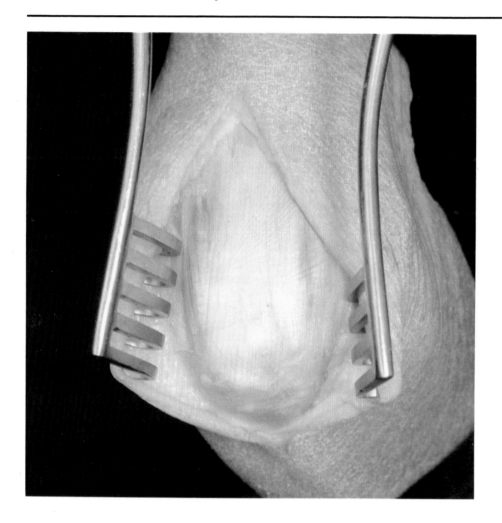

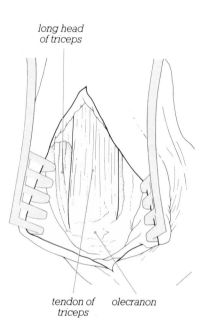

long head
of triceps

tendon of
triceps

olecranon

Fig. 10.3 A hole of a size appropriate to the fixing screw is drilled through the olecranon in the long axis of the ulna.

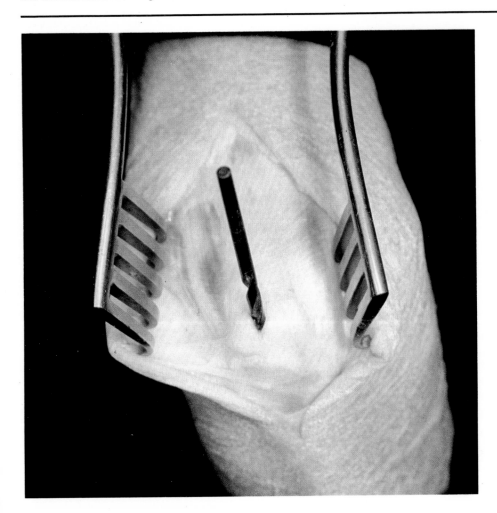

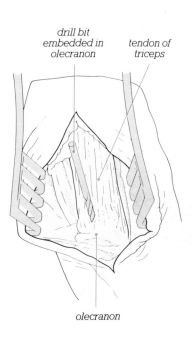

drill bit
embedded in
olecranon

tendon of
triceps

olecranon

Fig. 10.4 The fibres of the triceps tendon and the periosteum are divided transversely across the olecranon about 1–2cm distal to its tip.

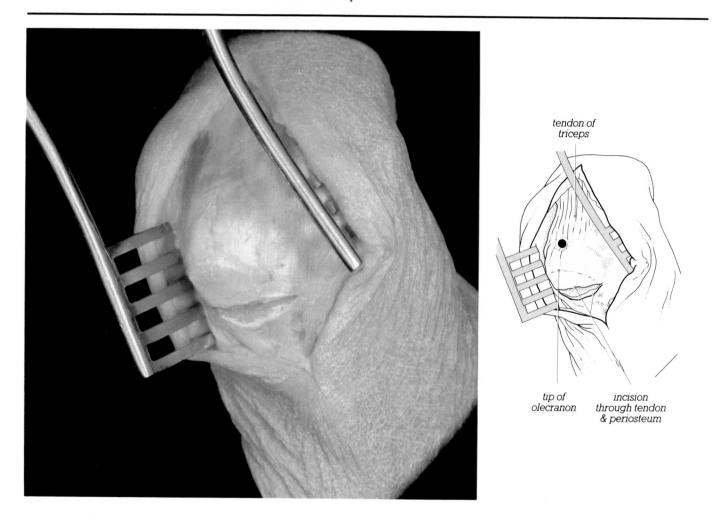

tendon of
triceps

tip of
olecranon

incision
through tendon
& periosteum

Fig. 10.5 The olecranon is divided at this level using either a sharp osteotome or an oscillating saw. The proximal fragment is retracted proximally on the triceps tendon to which it is still attached. The joint is closed with a long lag screw the size of the drilled hole.

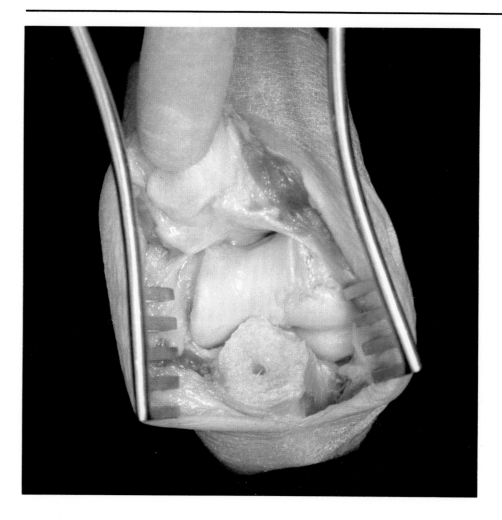

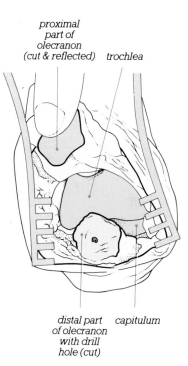

proximal
part of
olecranon
(cut & reflected)   trochlea

distal part   capitulum
of olecranon
with drill
hole (cut)

11 Exposure of the Common Flexor Origin and Ulnar Nerve at the Elbow (Right)

Fig. 11.1 The incision is centred over the medial epicondyle along the line of the ulnar nerve.

Points to consider

- The ulnar nerve is most easily located proximally. If it is not visible after the skin incision, it should be palpated where it lies in its groove.

- Careless dissection of the ulnar nerve may cut small branches to flexor carpi ulnaris.

- The intermuscular septum may kink the nerve in its displaced position and therefore should be divided proximally.

- Do not sew the nerve into the skin closure.

Position

The patient is supine with the arm abducted and externally rotated and the elbow flexed on a side table. A high tourniquet is applied.

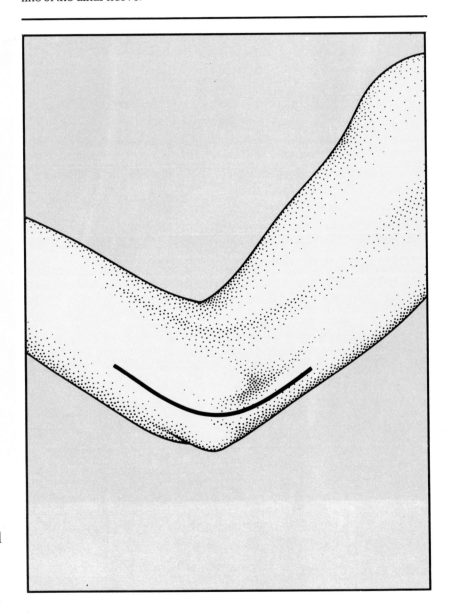

Fig. 11.2 The skin is retracted and the ulnar nerve located proximally.

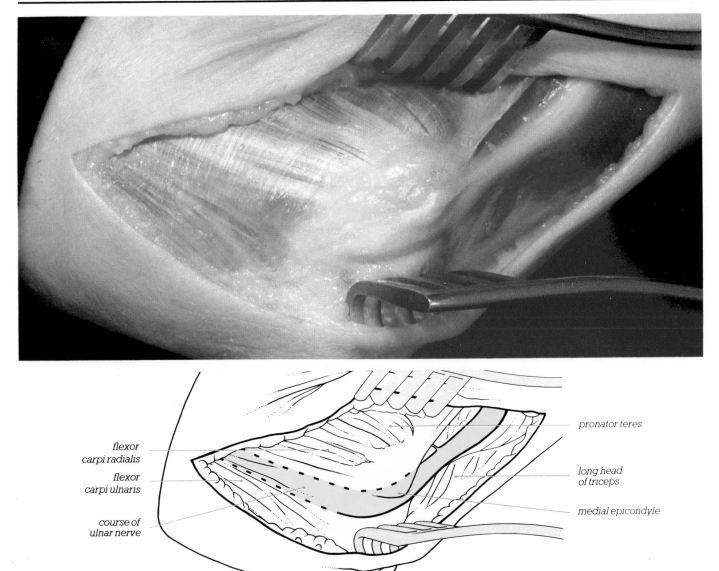

flexor carpi radialis

flexor carpi ulnaris

course of ulnar nerve

pronator teres

long head of triceps

medial epicondyle

Fig. 11.3 By incising the deep fascia and flexor carpi ulnaris the nerve is released from its bed. Several small branches are often seen; these branches can be dissected proximally from the main body of the nerve to allow the nerve to be displaced anteriorly. Once displaced, the nerve should lie comfortably. The nerve bed should be prepared proximally by dividing the medial intermuscular septum, which will allow greater freedom to reposition the nerve.

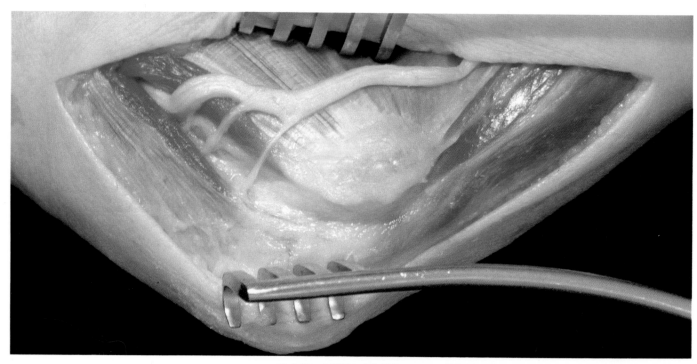

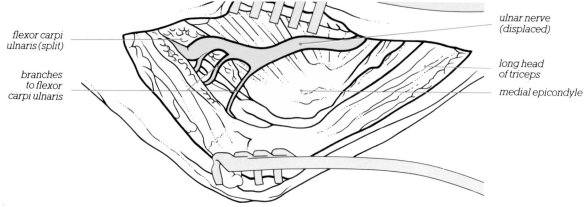

flexor carpi ulnaris (split)

branches to flexor carpi ulnaris

ulnar nerve (displaced)

long head of triceps

medial epicondyle

Fig. 11.4 Some surgeons prefer to cut a bed for the nerve in the muscles of the common flexor origin. The wound is closed, taking particular care not to transfix or ligate the nerve with the subcutaneous sutures.

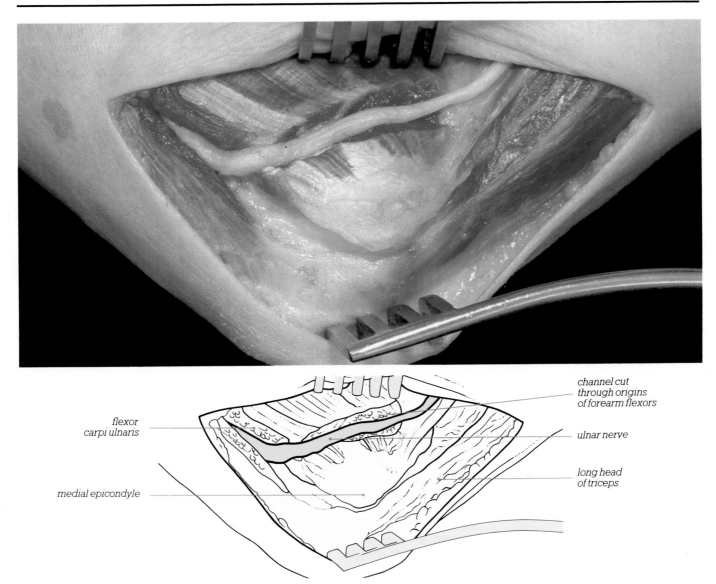

channel cut
through origins
of forearm flexors

flexor
carpi ulnaris

ulnar nerve

long head
of triceps

medial epicondyle

12 Exposure of the Radial Nerve at the Elbow (Right)

Fig. 12.1 The incision follows the line of the lateral supracondylar ridge to the lateral epicondyle of the humerus and runs over the bulk of the extensor muscles in the long axis of the forearm.

Points to consider

- Care must be taken not to damage the posterior interosseous nerve or the radial nerve during the retraction required for exposure.

Position

The patient is supine with the shoulder abducted and the limb on an arm board. The elbow is flexed at ninety degrees and the forearm pronated.

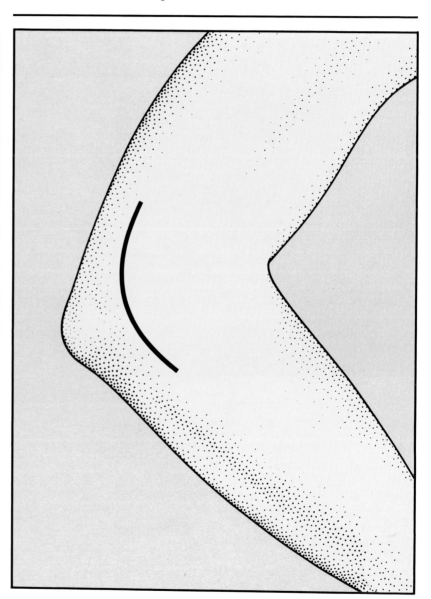

Fig. 12.2 Brachioradialis and extensor carpi radialis longus are identified and a plane developed between the medial border of brachioradialis and lateral border of brachialis.

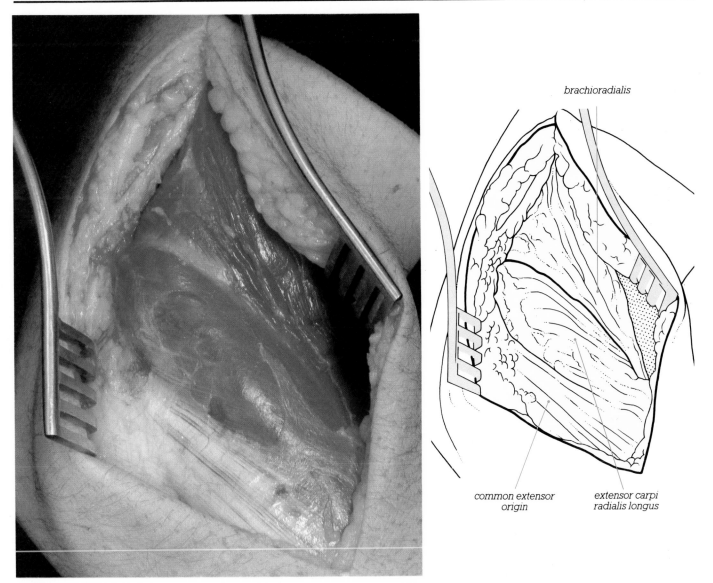

brachioradialis

common extensor origin

extensor carpi radialis longus

Fig. 12.3 The radial nerve runs under brachioradialis. The elbow is flexed further; dissection distally reveals the origin of the posterior interosseous nerve which runs under the aponeurotic fibres of extensor carpi radialis brevis towards supinator which it pierces.

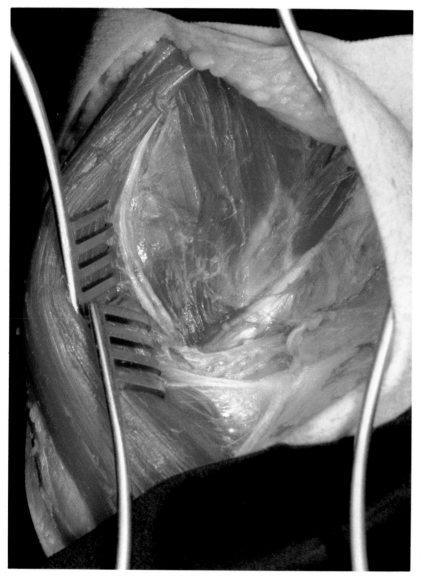

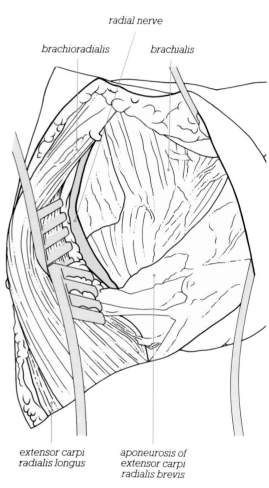

radial nerve

brachioradialis   brachialis

extensor carpi
radialis longus

aponeurosis of
extensor carpi
radialis brevis

13 Exposure of the Brachial Artery at the Elbow (Right)

Fig. 13.1 The S-shaped incision is centred on the elbow crease, commencing proximally on the medial side of the biceps tendon, running transversely across the elbow crease and distally over brachioradialis. The superficial veins are exposed and ligated.

Points to consider

- Careful dissection is required especially if the patient's pulse is weak or absent.

Position

The patient is supine with the limb abducted and fully supinated on an arm board. No tourniquet is applied.

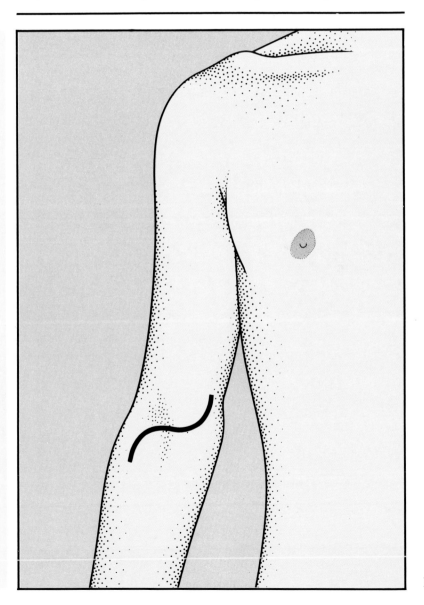

Fig. 13.2 The biceps tendon and aponeurosis are identified and, on its medial side, the brachial artery and median nerve are found, the nerve lying medially. The artery is dissected free of its accompanying veins and the median nerve.

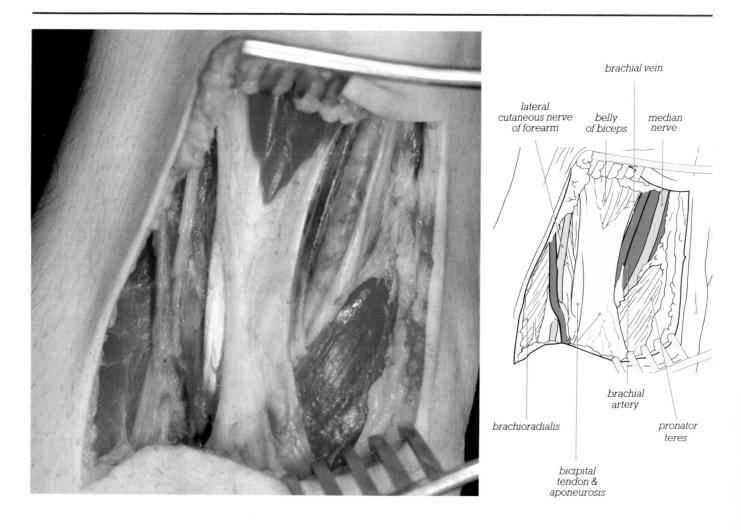

Fig. 13.3 Slings are applied around the artery and any branches. If access to the lumen is needed, a transverse arteriotomy is preferred.

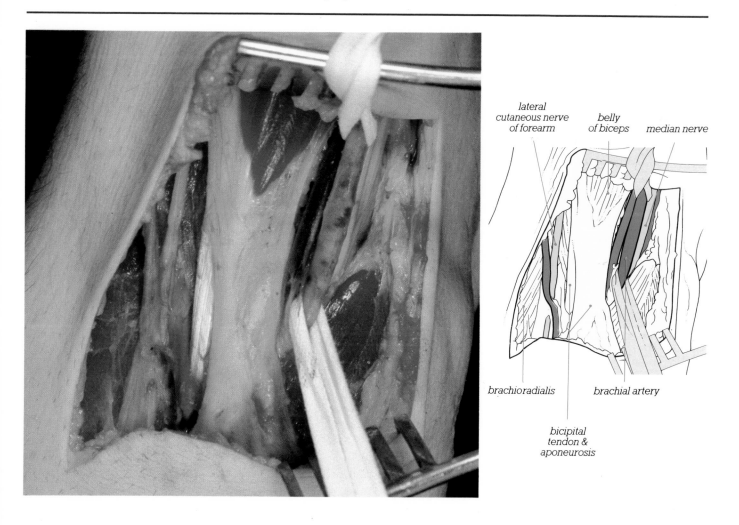

lateral
cutaneous nerve
of forearm

belly
of biceps

median nerve

brachioradialis

brachial artery

bicipital
tendon &
aponeurosis

14 Exposure of the Radial Head (Right)

Fig. 14.1 The 10cm L-shaped incision runs in the line of the lower humeral shaft and around the posterior aspect of the lateral epicondyle, continuing in line with the radial shaft.

Points to consider

- The orbicular ligament can be retracted and should be preserved if possible.

- The greatest hazard of this incision is damage to the posterior interosseous nerve lying within the body of supinator. Great care should be exercised when dissecting distally which, for safety, should be avoided.

Position
The patient is supine with the arm on a side table, the elbow flexed with the lateral aspect superior or, alternatively, with the arm held across the chest. A tourniquet is applied.

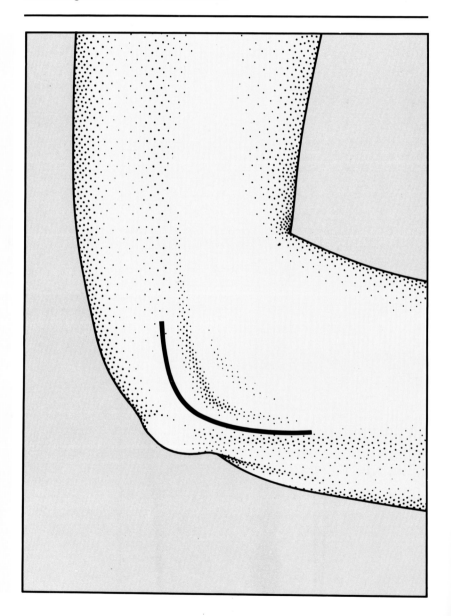

Fig. 14.2 The lateral epicondyle and common extensor origin are identified. (If a lateral release for 'tennis elbow' were being performed, the latter would be detached from its bony origin.) The extensor muscles are incised across the line of the fibres.

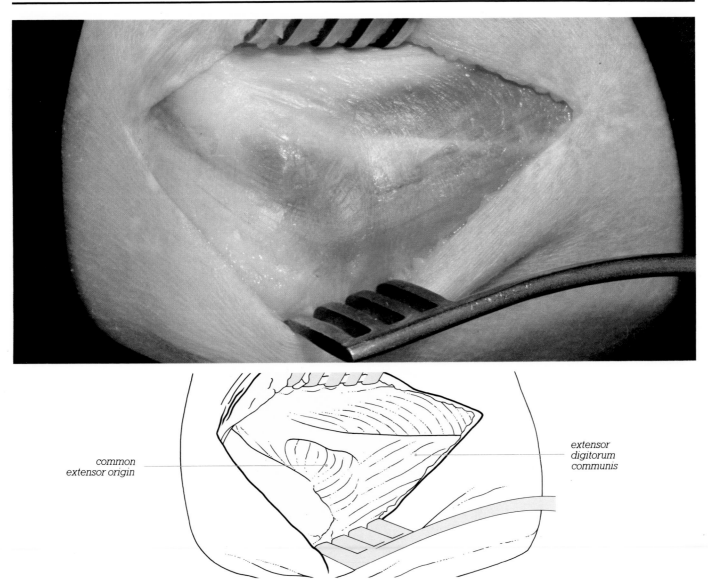

common extensor origin

extensor digitorum communis

Fig. 14.3 Incision through the joint capsule and synovium will expose the capitulum and the radial head.

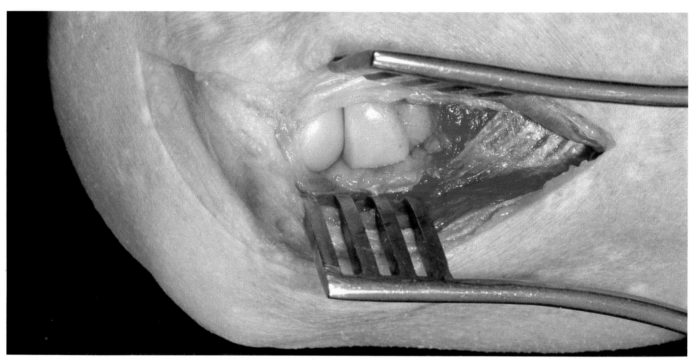

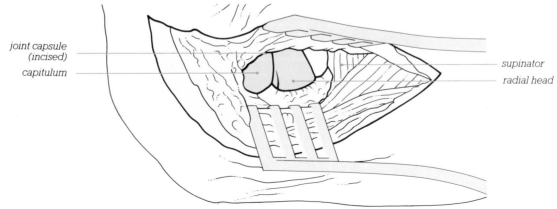

joint capsule (incised)

capitulum

supinator

radial head

Fig. 14.4 The capsular incision can be extended distally to expose the entire radial head. Great care should be taken when dividing supinator, which is normally not necessary, that the posterior interosseous nerve is not divided.

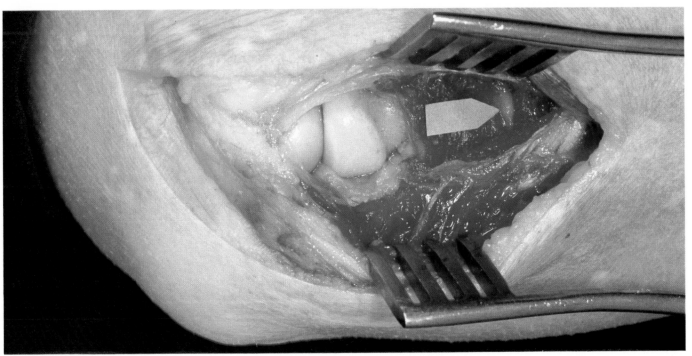

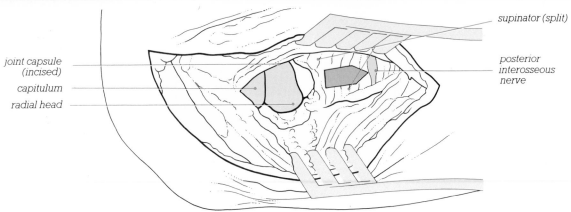

joint capsule (incised)

capitulum

radial head

supinator (split)

posterior interosseous nerve

15 Anterior Approach to the Shaft of the Radius (Left)

Fig. 15.1 The incision commences lateral to the biceps tendon in the antecubital fossa and curves medially along the edge of brachioradialis towards the radial styloid process.

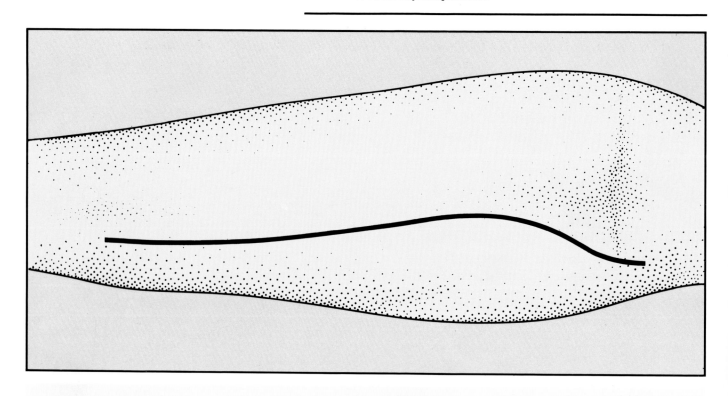

Points to consider

- The distal third of the radius may be reached by using the lower part of this incision, but approaches to the proximal radius must include identification of supinator and the vulnerable posterior interosseous nerve.

Position

The patient is supine, the limb on an arm table. A tourniquet is applied to the upper arm.

Fig. 15.2 Superficial veins are tied and the deep fascia divided in the same line as the skin. Brachioradialis and extensor carpi radialis longus and brevis are retracted as one unit, using blunt dissection from the lateral side of the biceps tendon and moving distally. A leash of recurrent radial vessels is identified, tied and divided.

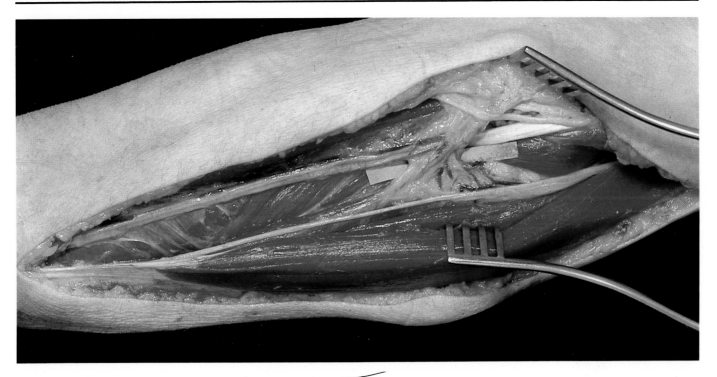

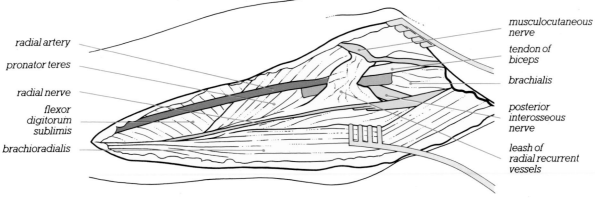

radial artery

pronator teres

radial nerve

flexor digitorum sublimis

brachioradialis

musculocutaneous nerve

tendon of biceps

brachialis

posterior interosseous nerve

leash of radial recurrent vessels

1.61

Fig. 15.3 Supinator is exposed by retraction of the wad of three muscles which may require brachioradialis to be detached from the radial styloid process and the elbow flexed. The radial nerve, with the posterior interosseous branch piercing supinator, can now be seen.

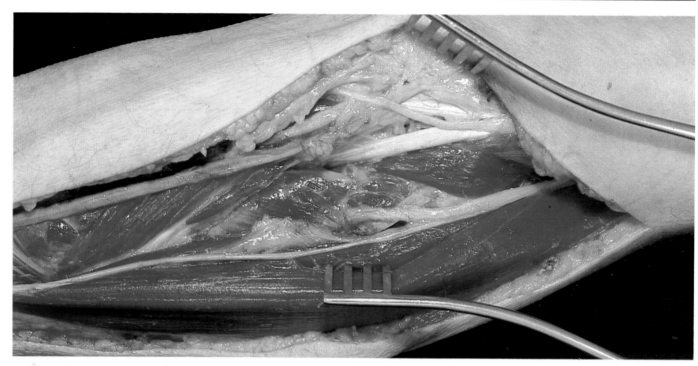

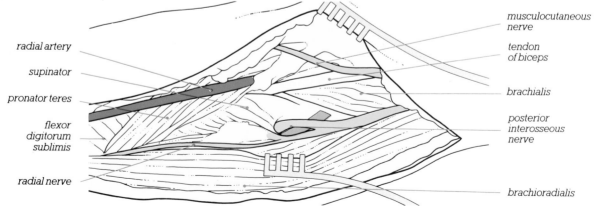

musculocutaneous nerve

tendon of biceps

brachialis

posterior interosseous nerve

brachioradialis

radial artery

supinator

pronator teres

flexor digitorum sublimis

radial nerve

Fig. 15.4 Supinator, which contains and protects the posterior interosseous nerve, is detached from the radius by cutting onto the bone immediately lateral to the biceps tendon. Using a periosteal elevator, supinator and the periosteum are reflected from the radius. Dissection is continued between the radial nerve and artery along the length of the radius. Pronation of the forearm will increase exposure of the bone.

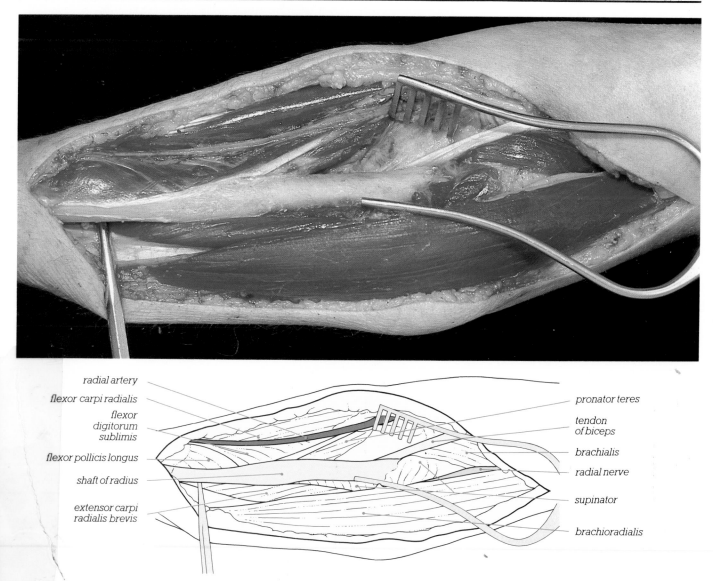

radial artery

flexor carpi radialis

flexor digitorum sublimis

flexor pollicis longus

shaft of radius

extensor carpi radialis brevis

pronator teres

tendon of biceps

brachialis

radial nerve

supinator

brachioradialis

16 Approach to the Ventral Aspect of the Distal Radius (Right)

Fig. 16.1 The longitudinal incision is over the ventral aspect of the radius between the palpable tendon of flexor carpi radialis and the radial artery and extends distally to the joint crease.

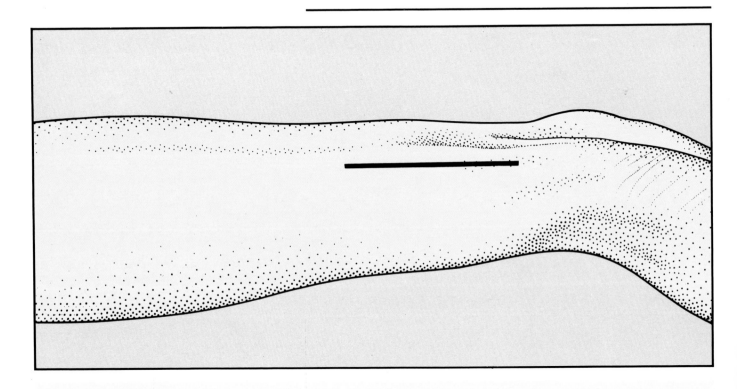

Points to consider

- This incision is suitable for the application of a buttress plate, for example, in the treatment of a Smith's fracture.

- It is useful to identify the radial pulse at the wrist before the tourniquet is inflated.

Position
The patient is supine with the arm supinated on an additional table. A tourniquet is applied.

Fig. 16.2 The incision is deepened and the tendon of flexor carpi radialis and the tendon and belly of flexor pollicis longus identified.

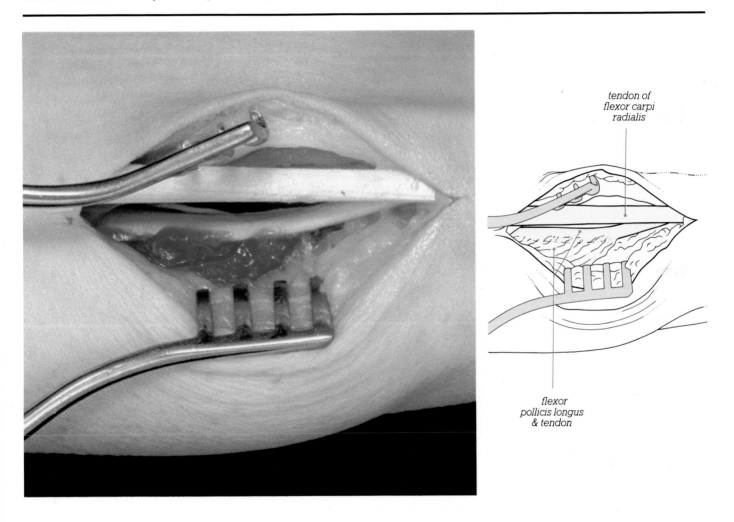

tendon of
flexor carpi
radialis

flexor
pollicis longus
& tendon

Fig. 16.3 The two tendons are separated. The median nerve is protected by flexor carpi radialis and the radial artery by flexor pollicis longus. Pronator quadratus is lifted from the radius with a periosteal elevator to reveal the ventral aspect of the distal radius.

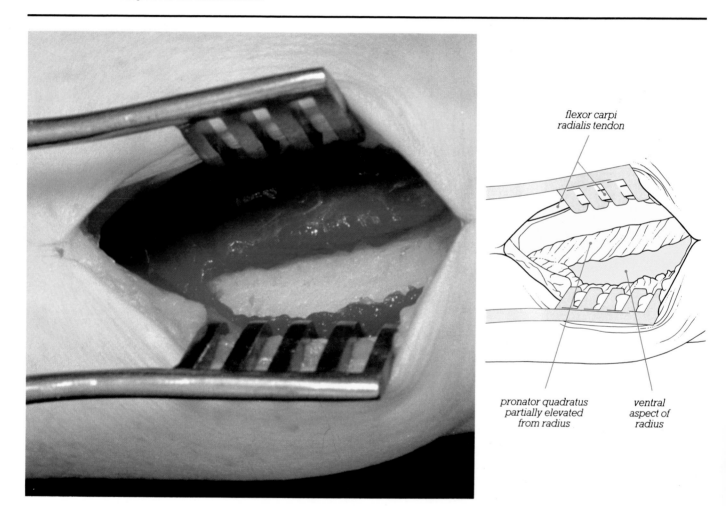

flexor carpi
radialis tendon

pronator quadratus
partially elevated
from radius

ventral
aspect of
radius

17 Approach to the Shaft of the Ulna (Right)

Fig. 17.1 The incision extends from the olecranon to the ulnar styloid process along the subcutaneous border of the bone.

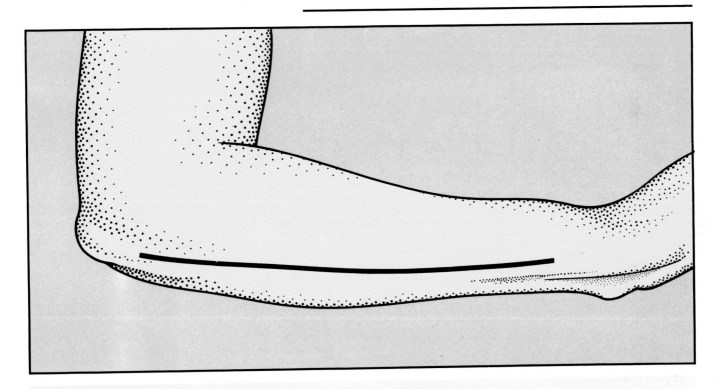

Points to consider

- This exposure of the ulna is very simple and safe, providing that the incision is made along the subcutaneous part of the bone at the elbow and wrist. It is important to maintain this relationship.

Position

The patient is supine with the arm over the chest or pronated on a side table. A tourniquet is applied.

Fig. 17.2 The aponeurosis of flexor carpi ulnaris and extensor carpi ulnaris are identified. An incision is made between the two down to the bone.

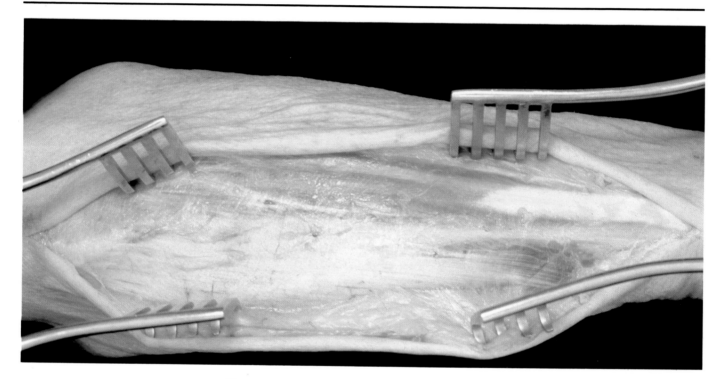

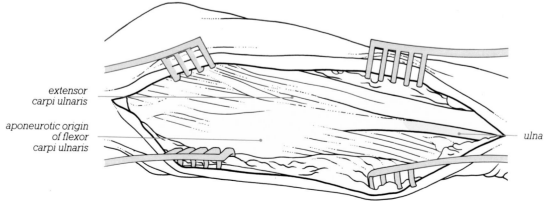

extensor
carpi ulnaris

aponeurotic origin
of flexor
carpi ulnaris

ulna

Fig. 17.3 Using a periosteal elevator, the belly of flexor digitorum profundus, which lies beneath the aponeurosis of flexor carpi ulnaris, is reflected to expose the ulnar shaft.

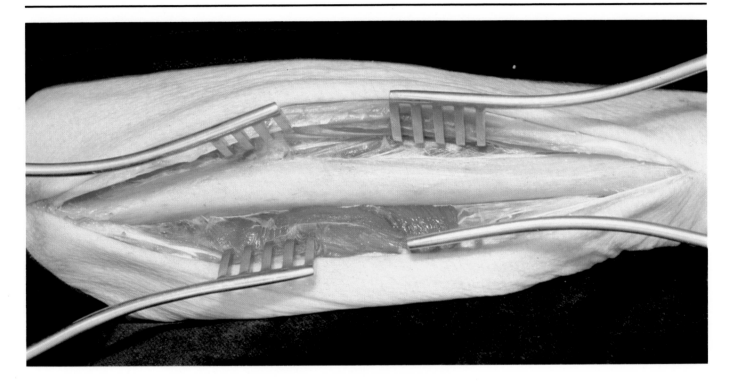

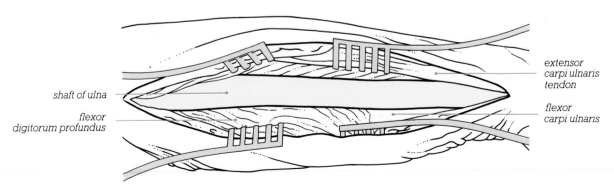

shaft of ulna

flexor
digitorum profundus

extensor
carpi ulnaris
tendon

flexor
carpi ulnaris

18 Exposure of the Radial Artery and Cephalic Vein at the Wrist (Left)

Fig. 18.1 The incision is over the distal 5cm of the radius between the cephalic vein and the palpable radial artery.

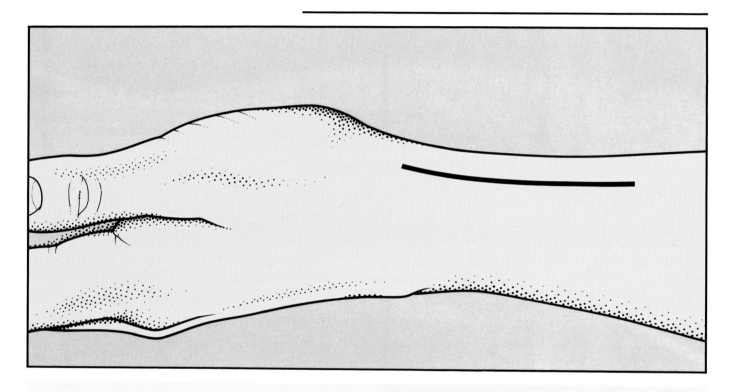

Points to consider

- If this incision is being used to form a fistula between the cephalic vein and radial artery, it is essential to first determine if the ulnar artery is patent.

- The incision may have to be extended to give suitable exposure of the vessels.

Position

The patient is supine with the arm abducted and supinated on a hand table. No tourniquet is applied.

Fig. 18.2 The radial artery and cephalic vein are exposed and dissected free. Branches and tributaries are ligated and divided to allow the two vessels to be approximated without tension.

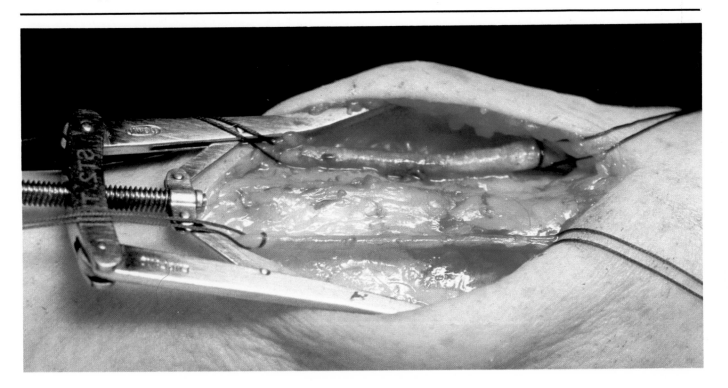

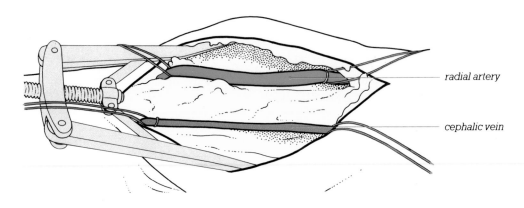

radial artery

cephalic vein

19 Approach to the Carpal Scaphoid (Left)

Fig. 19.1 The slightly curved incision extends from the base of the second metacarpal along the distal end of the radius.

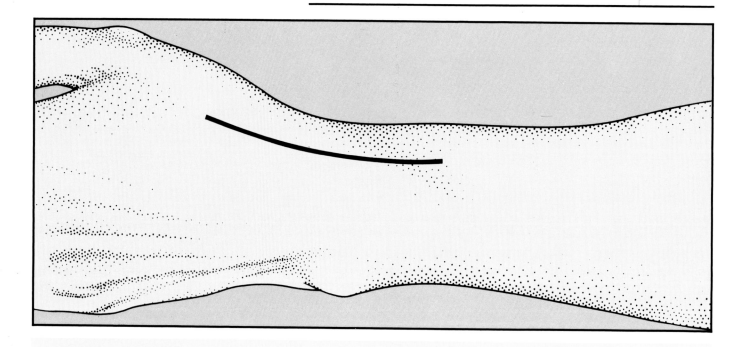

Points to consider

- If the superficial branches of the radial nerve are divided or damaged, a painful neuroma may result.

- Manipulation of the wrist joint allows easier identification and exposure of the scaphoid.

- It is recommended that the tourniquet be released before closure of the wound to reveal any damage to the radial artery. If absolutely necessary the radial artery can be tied, but it is advisable to avoid this. It should also be confirmed that there is an adequate ulnar arterial supply to the hand.

Position

The patient is supine with the arm abducted and pronated on a hand table. A tourniquet is applied after exsanguination of the limb.

Fig. 19.2 Superficial veins are tied or retracted. Fibres of the superficial branch of the radial nerve are identified and retracted.

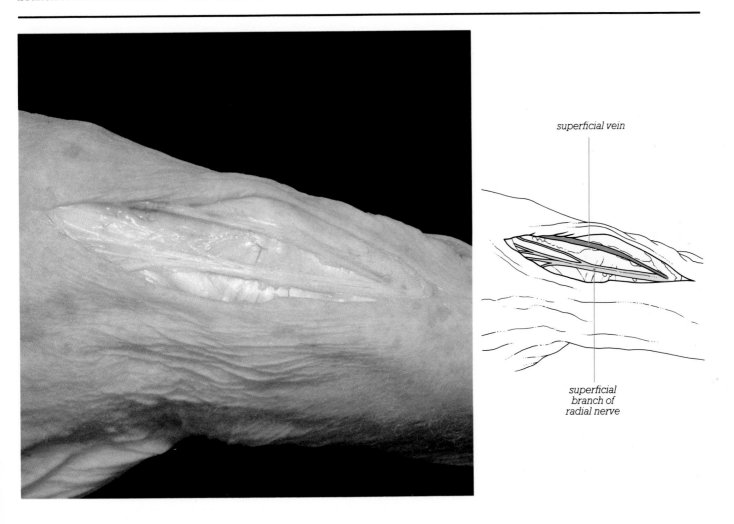

superficial vein

superficial branch of radial nerve

Fig. 19.3 Dissection is deepened to define the 'anatomical snuff box' between the tendons of extensor pollicis longus and extensor carpi radialis longus on one border, and abductor pollicis longus and extensor pollicis brevis on the other.

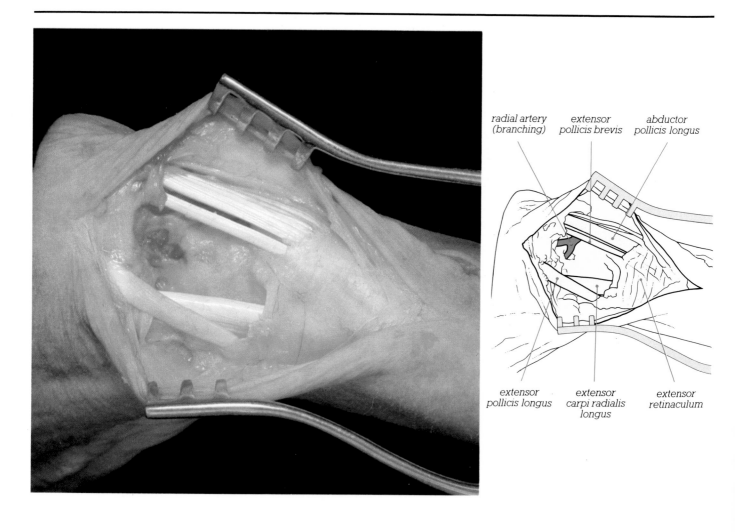

Fig. 19.4   The lateral edge of the scaphoid is then revealed; the radial artery may require retraction to give a better view.

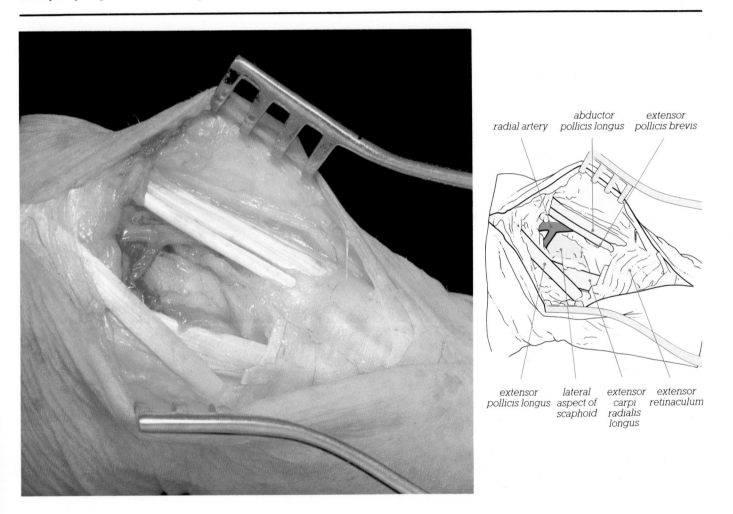

radial artery | abductor pollicis longus | extensor pollicis brevis

extensor pollicis longus | lateral aspect of scaphoid | extensor carpi radialis longus | extensor retinaculum

20 Approach to the Wrist Joint (Left)

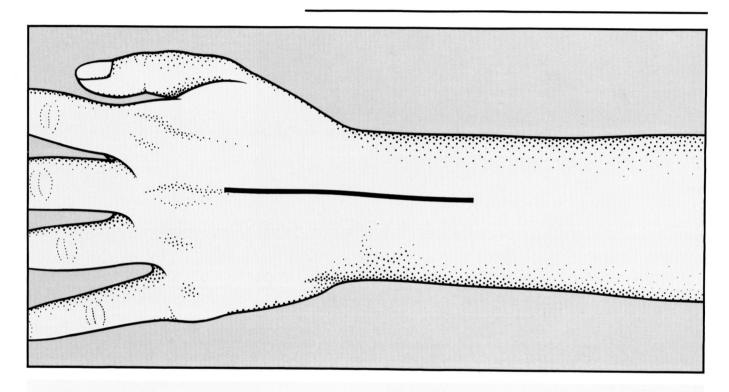

Points to consider

- If this incision is performed for arthrodesis of the joint, a donor site for the bone graft will be required.

Position
The limb is prone on an arm table with a tourniquet applied.

Fig. 20.2 Cutaneous nerves are preserved where possible and the extensor retinaculum identified and divided in the long axis of the wrist.

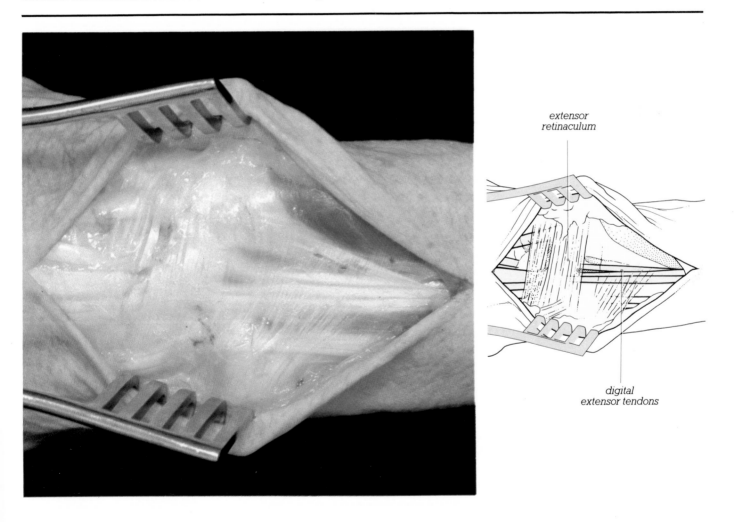

extensor
retinaculum

digital
extensor tendons

Fig. 20.3 The extensor tendons are freed and retracted laterally (towards the ulna).

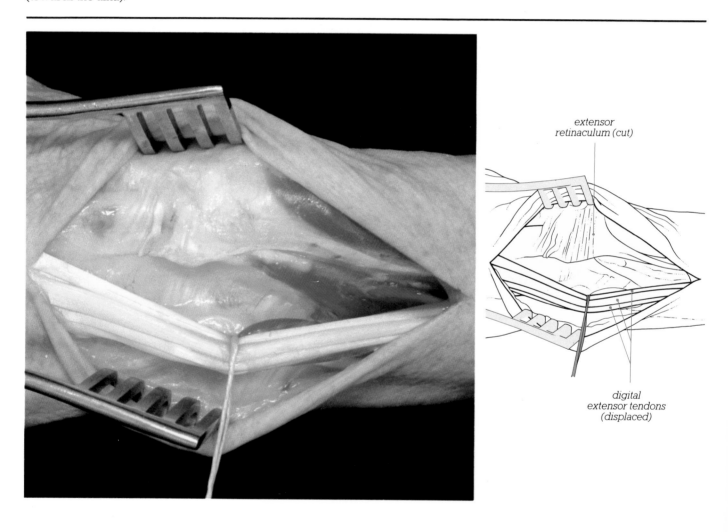

extensor
retinaculum (cut)

digital
extensor tendons
(displaced)

Fig. 20.4 The joint capsules are incised over the radiocarpal, intercarpal and carpometacarpal joints.

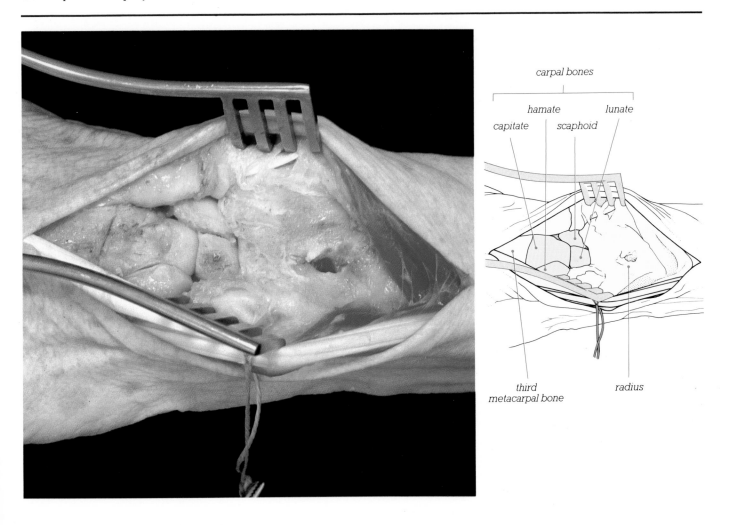

carpal bones

hamate   lunate

capitate   scaphoid

third metacarpal bone   radius

21 de Quervain's Release (Right)

Fig. 21.1 The 2cm transverse incision is only skin-deep across the radial styloid process.

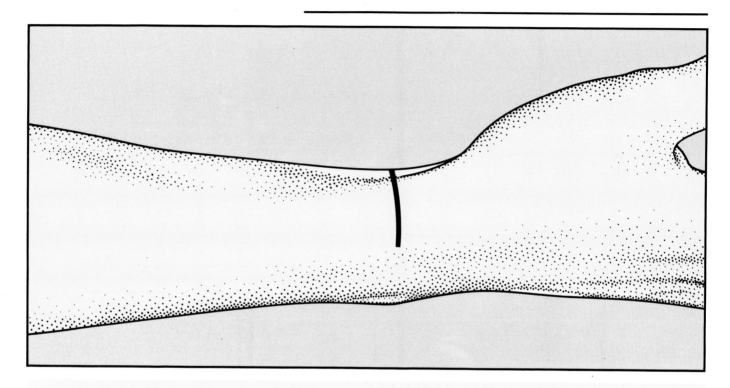

Points to consider

- Extensor pollicis brevis occurs occasionally in a separate sheath which must be divided.

- In the initial part of the dissection, preservation of the small branches of the radial nerve is important.

Position
The patient is supine with the limb on an arm table, a tourniquet applied and the radial border of the hand uppermost.

Fig. 21.2 Small branches of the radial nerve are identified and preserved.

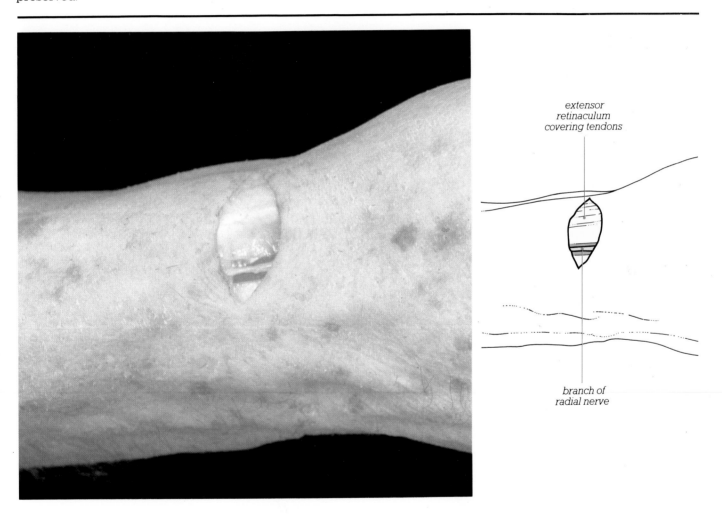

extensor
retinaculum
covering tendons

branch of
radial nerve

Fig. 21.3 Dissecting through the fat, a small transverse incision is made in the extensor retinaculum to identify the paired tendons of extensor pollicis brevis and abductor pollicis longus.

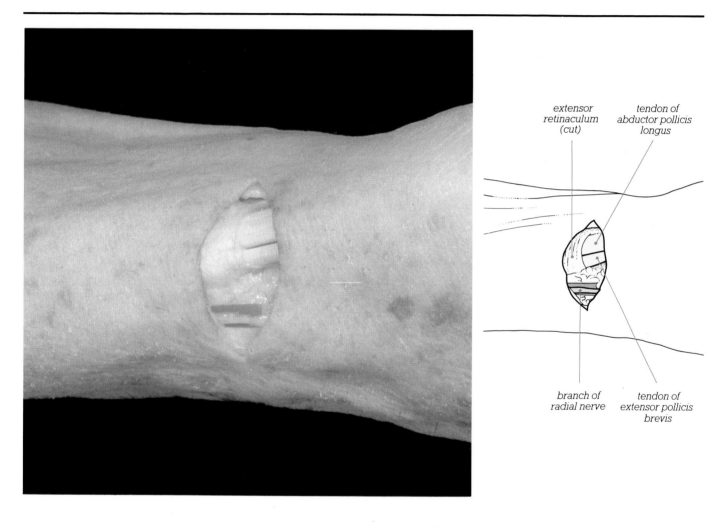

extensor
retinaculum
(cut)

tendon of
abductor pollicis
longus

branch of
radial nerve

tendon of
extensor pollicis
brevis

Fig. 21.4 The extensor retinaculum is incised in line with the tendons to divide the thickened tendon sheaths distally and proximally.

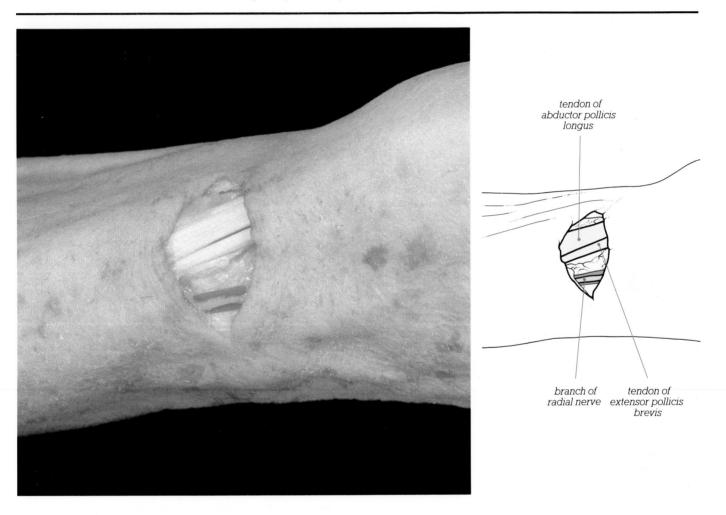

tendon of
abductor pollicis
longus

branch of
radial nerve

tendon of
extensor pollicis
brevis

22 Carpal Tunnel Decompression (Left)

Fig. 22.1 The incision can be up to 5cm long. It commences medial to the thenar skin crease just distal to the flexor crease of the wrist and extends distally into the palm.

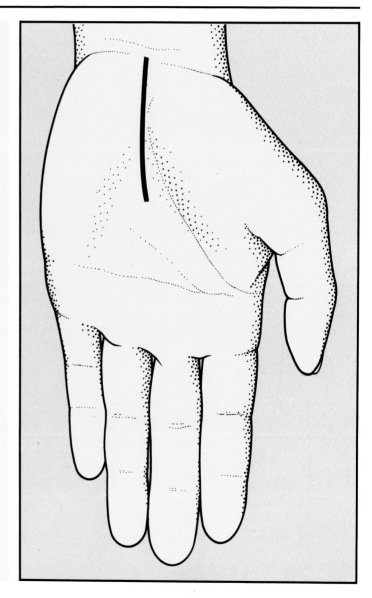

Points to consider

- If the hand is not fully supinated, dissection will easily be oblique towards the ulna instead of at right angles to the palm.

- When the retinaculum is divided completely, the cut edges spring apart and lie parallel to each other. If division is incomplete, the cut edges approximate to each other at one end.

- Incomplete division either proximally or distally beyond the incision can be palpated using the curved part of the McDonald dissector as a probe.

- The nerve should lie free at the end of the procedure. If the epimysium appears to be tight, this may be split longitudinally. Ganglia or thickened synovium should be removed.

- Closure of the skin only is required to end the procedure.

Position

The patient is supine with the limb on an arm board and a tourniquet applied. The hand should be fully supinated. A lead hand may be used to maintain this position during surgery.

Fig. 22.2 The incision is deepened through the palmar fat until the flexor retinaculum is identified.

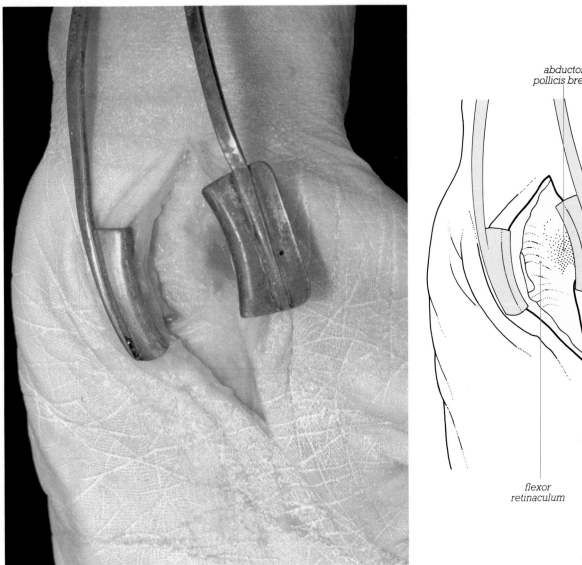

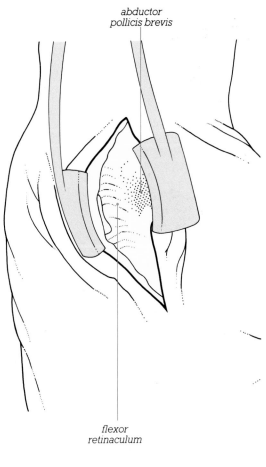

abductor
pollicis brevis

flexor
retinaculum

CARPAL TUNNEL DECOMPRESSION (LEFT)

Fig. 22.3 In the same line and at ninety degrees to the palm, the flexor retinaculum is incised until there is complete division but over a very short length. A McDonald dissector is introduced through this small hole and placed over the median nerve. The retinaculum is then divided over its entire length while the nerve lies safely beneath the dissector. The retinaculum and deep fascia should be divided for a distance of 2cm proximal to the distal wrist crease and distal to the superficial palmar arch vessels.

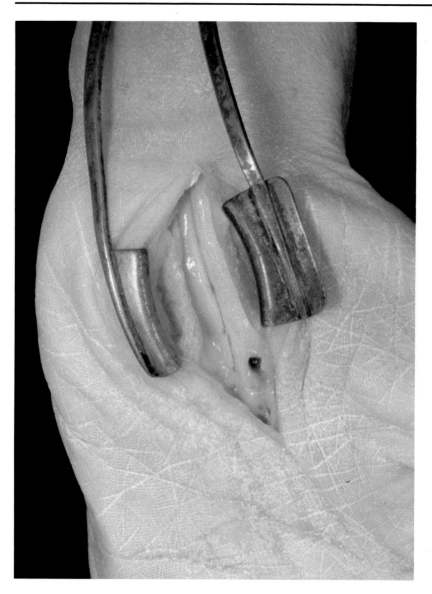

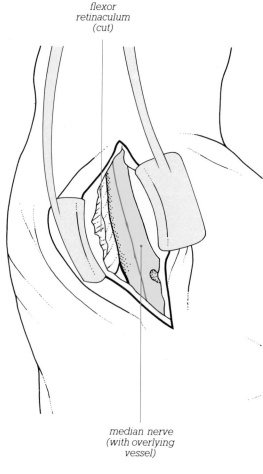

flexor
retinaculum
(cut)

median nerve
(with overlying
vessel)

Fig. 22.4 Dissection should be maintained in the long axis of the hand. To stray laterally would jeopardize the recurrent motor branch to the thenar muscle.

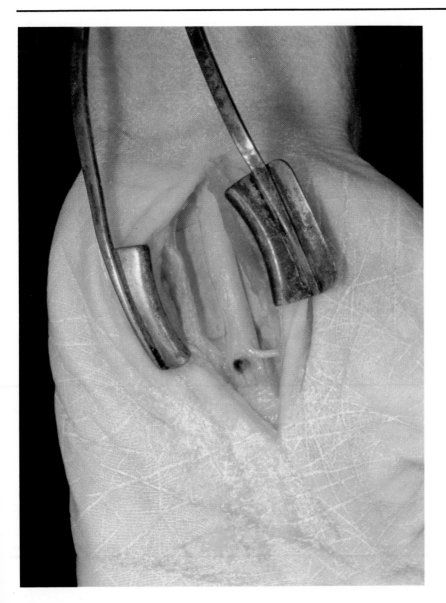

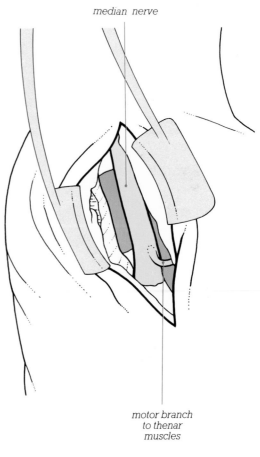

median nerve

motor branch
to thenar
muscles

2 Exposures of the Lower Limb

23 Anterolateral Approach to the Hip Joint (Left)

Fig. 23.1 The incision runs from the anterior superior iliac spine to the greater trochanter where it curves to run down the lateral aspect of the femur.

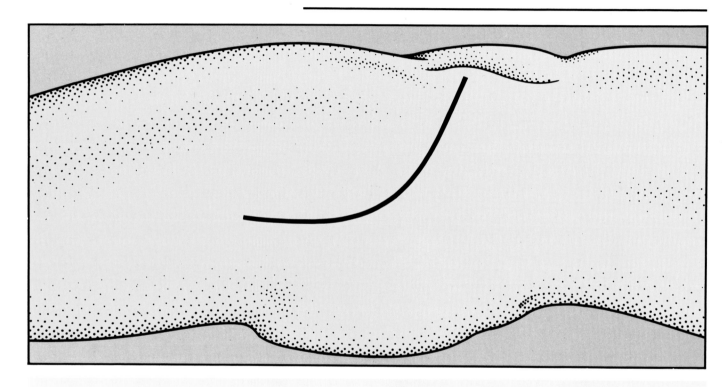

Points to consider

- The two limbs of the skin incision should be joined not by a sharp angle but by a curve.

- A wider exposure can be obtained by detaching the anterior one-third of the gluteus medius tendon from the greater trochanter.

Position

The patient is supine with a sandbag under the affected hip. Draping allows full movement of the hip and knee.

Fig. 23.2 The fascia lata and tensor fasciae latae are identified.

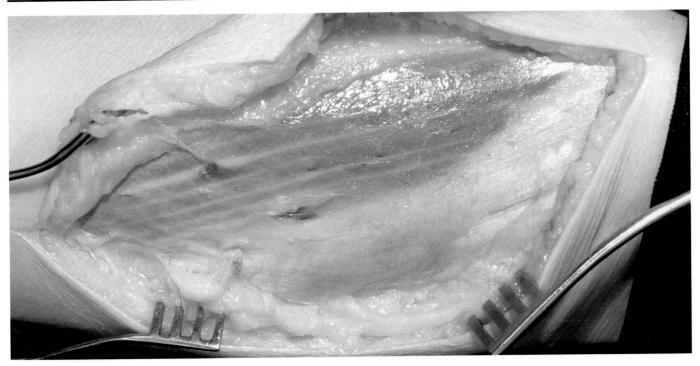

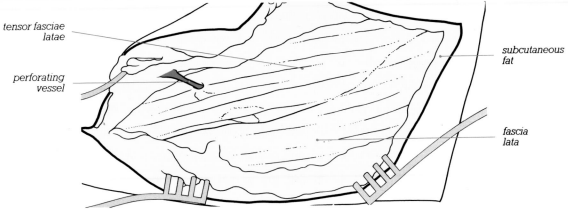

tensor fasciae
latae

perforating
vessel

subcutaneous
fat

fascia
lata

Fig. 23.3 The fascia lata is incised from just behind tensor fasciae latae to the greater trochanter. Tensor fasciae latae is reflected anteriorly, revealing the anterior border of gluteus medius which is retracted posteriorly. The incision in the fascia lata is extended distally along the lateral margin of the femoral shaft.

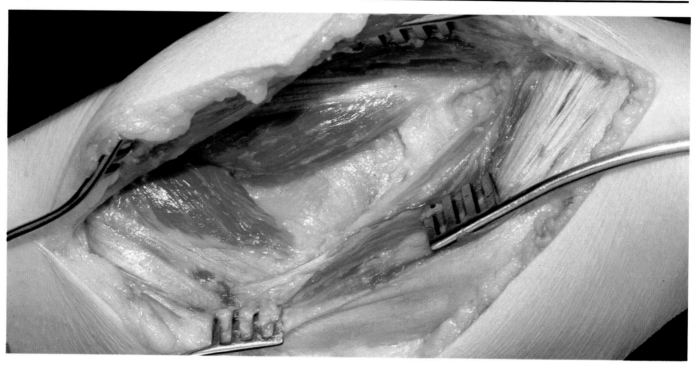

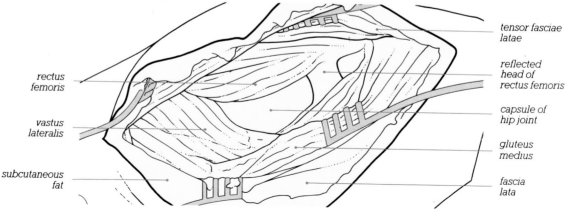

rectus femoris

vastus lateralis

subcutaneous fat

tensor fasciae latae

reflected head of rectus femoris

capsule of hip joint

gluteus medius

fascia lata

Fig. 23.4 Rectus femoris is retracted medially and the capsule of the hip joint incised in the line of the neck of the femur.

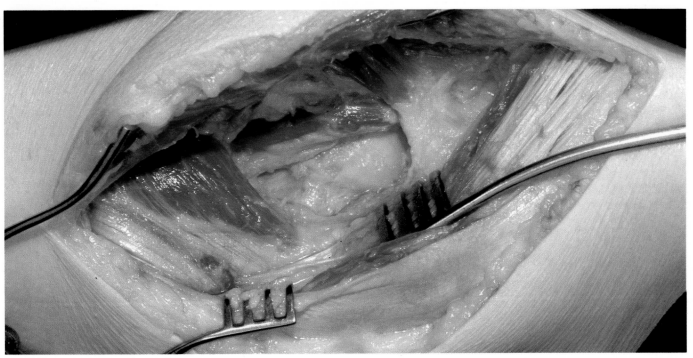

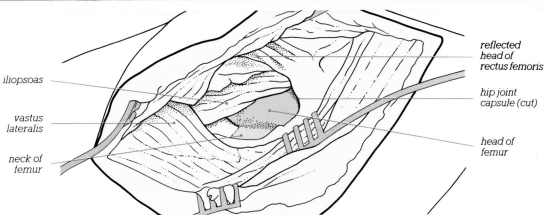

iliopsoas

vastus
lateralis

neck of
femur

reflected
head of
rectus femoris

hip joint
capsule (cut)

head of
femur

Fig. 23.5 To dislocate the femoral head it may be necessary to cut the reflected head of rectus femoris, as demonstrated in this specimen.

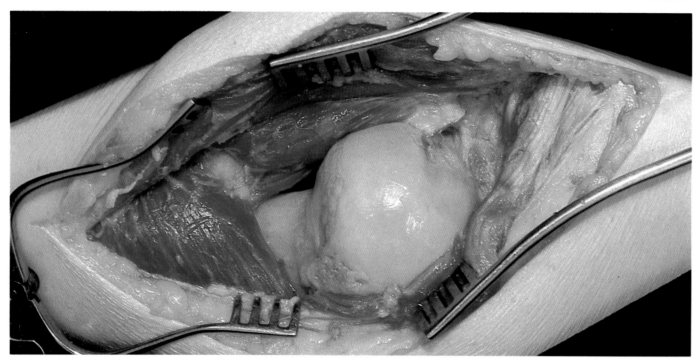

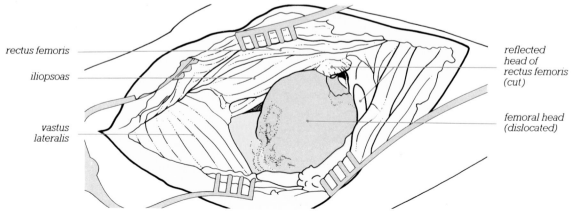

rectus femoris

iliopsoas

vastus lateralis

reflected head of rectus femoris (cut)

femoral head (dislocated)

Lateral Approach to the Hip Joint (Right)

Fig. 24.1 The incision is centred on the greater trochanter of the femur, extends downwards in the line of the shaft and curves posteriorly proximally.

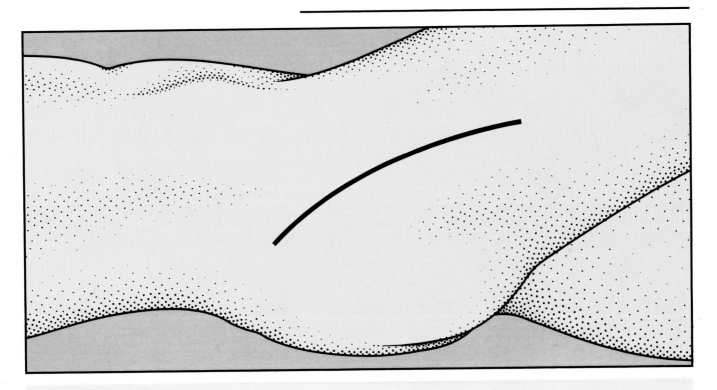

Points to consider

- If the incision is not centred on the greater trochanter but is too far anterior, a relieving incision may be necessary in the fascia lata.

- Incising the hip joint capsule allows safe intra-articular passage for the forceps and the saw.

- The position of the sciatic nerve must be confirmed before dividing the greater trochanter.

Position

The patient is supine with a small sandbag under the buttock.

Fig. 24.2 Continuing in the same line as the incision, the fascia lata is incised over the midlateral aspect of the trochanter and split in the line of its fibres.

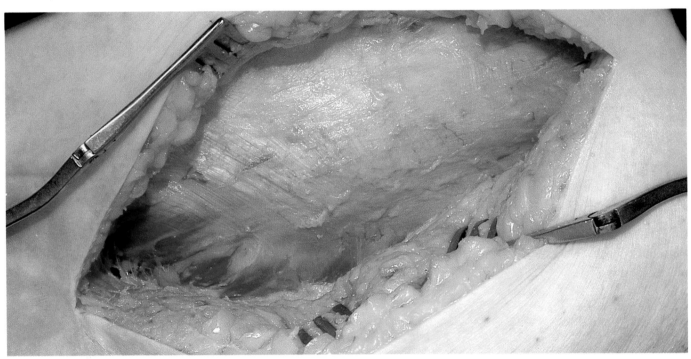

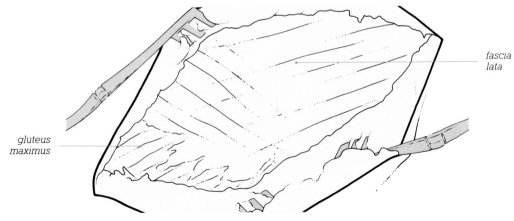

gluteus
maximus

fascia
lata

Fig. 24.3 The fascia lata is retracted, revealing the space between gluteus medius and vastus lateralis through which the capsule of the hip joint is divided. A pair of large curved forceps is passed round the superior aspect of the neck of the femur to emerge posterior to the trochanter.

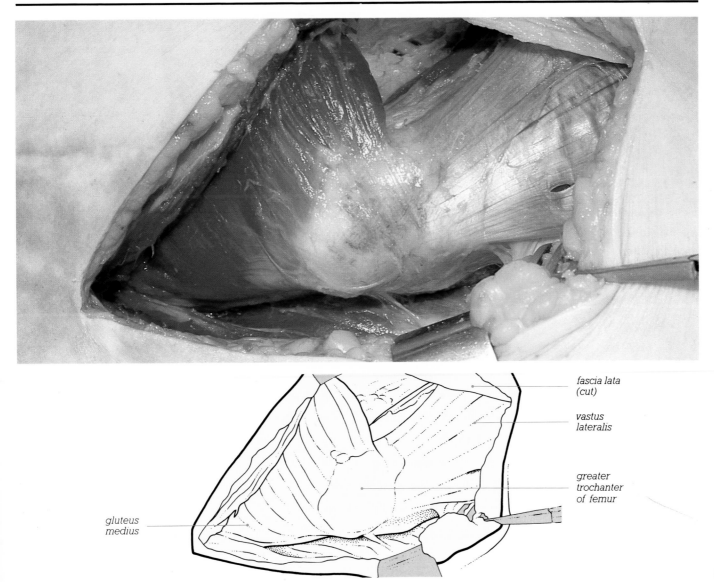

fascia lata (cut)

vastus lateralis

greater trochanter of femur

gluteus medius

2.9

Fig. 24.4 After checking that the sciatic nerve is free, the forceps are used to introduce a Gigli wire saw. Cutting in the line of the femoral neck, the greater trochanter is divided and retracted.

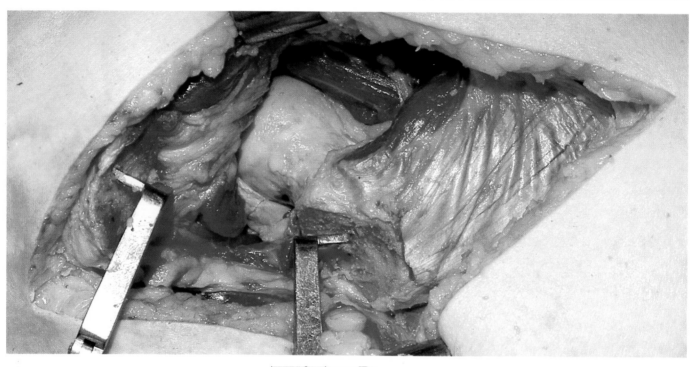

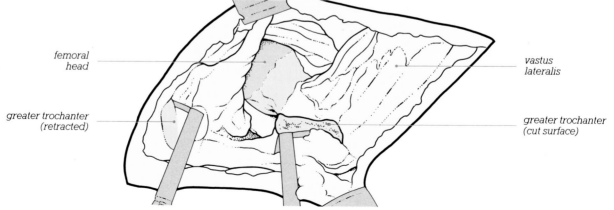

femoral
head

vastus
lateralis

greater trochanter
(retracted)

greater trochanter
(cut surface)

Fig. 24.5 The remaining capsule is trimmed and the hip dislocated by adduction, flexion and external rotation.

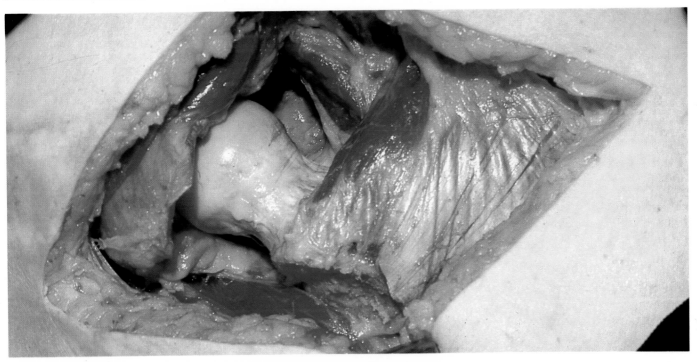

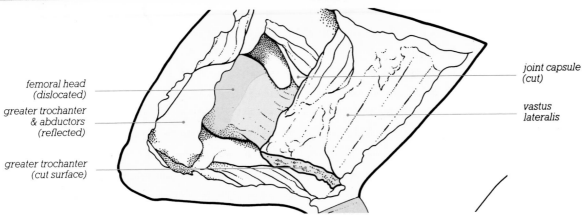

femoral head
(dislocated)

greater trochanter
& abductors
(reflected)

greater trochanter
(cut surface)

joint capsule
(cut)

vastus
lateralis

Fig. 24.6 The femoral neck is divided at an angle appropriate to the procedure, resulting in an excellent view of the acetabulum and the femoral canal.

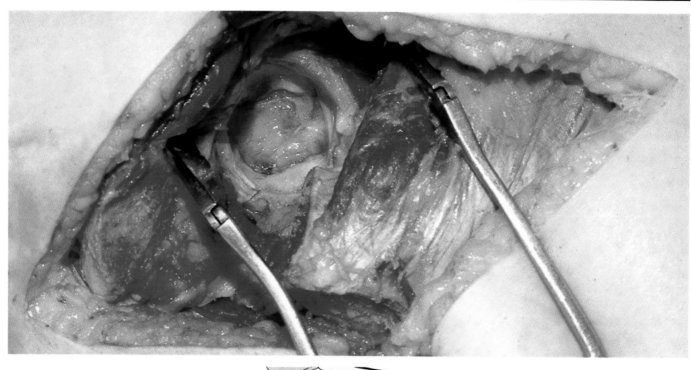

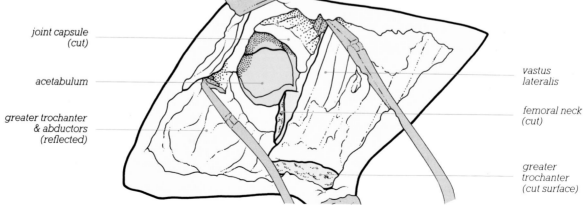

joint capsule
(cut)

acetabulum

greater trochanter
& abductors
(reflected)

vastus
lateralis

femoral neck
(cut)

greater
trochanter
(cut surface)

Posterior Approach to the Hip Joint (Right)

Fig. 25.1 The incision runs along the lateral aspect of the femur to the greater trochanter where it curves posteriorly towards the posterior superior iliac spine.

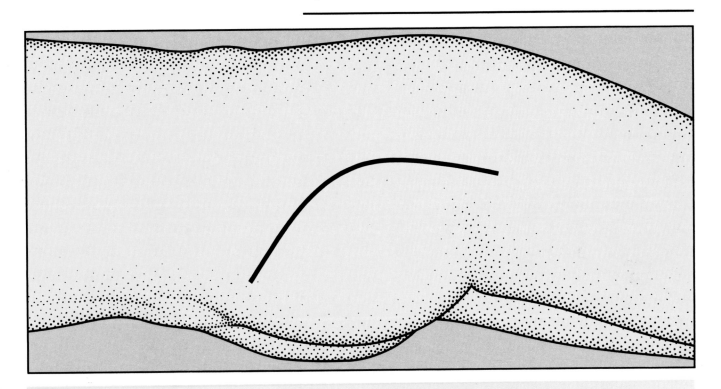

Points to consider
- The sciatic nerve need not be dissected free, but one should always be aware of its position and vulnerability.

- Posterior dislocation of the femoral head is not uncommon as a postoperative complication of this approach, so it is wise to detach only obturator internus and the gemelli to achieve dislocation at operation.

The additional detachment of piriformis superiorly and quadratus femoris inferiorly will produce a less stable hip postoperatively.

Position
The patient is placed on the sound side, supported by anterior and posterior cushions. Draping allows full movement of the affected hip and knee.

Fig. 25.2 The fascia lata and gluteus maximus are exposed.

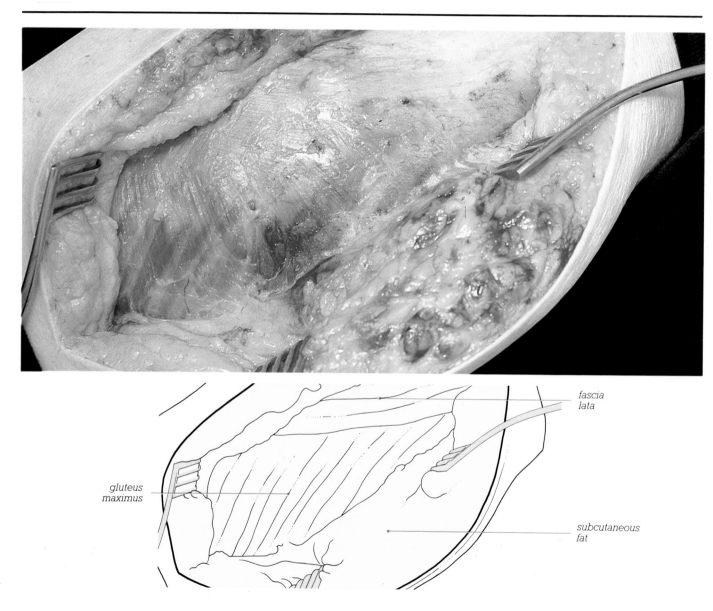

fascia
lata

gluteus
maximus

subcutaneous
fat

Fig. 25.3 The dissection is deepened in the line of the incision. The fascia lata is split along the lateral edge of the femur and gluteus maximus is split in the line of its fibres towards the posterior superior iliac spine.

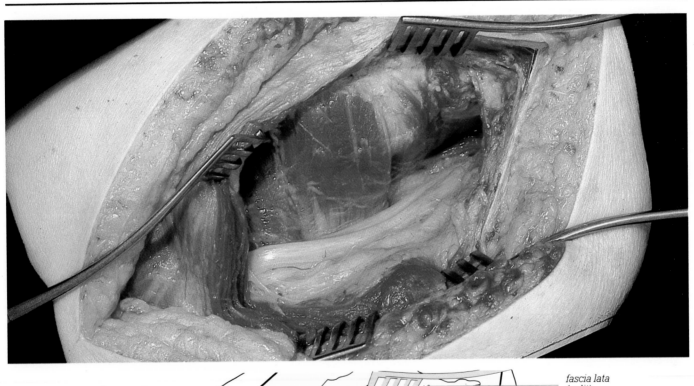

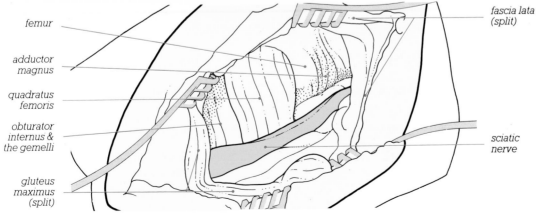

femur

adductor magnus

quadratus femoris

obturator internus & the gemelli

gluteus maximus (split)

fascia lata (split)

sciatic nerve

2.15

Fig. 25.4 The short rotators are detached from the trochanter. For clarity in this specimen, quadratus femoris is cut, but this should not normally be necessary. The capsule of the hip joint is incised in the line of the neck of the femur, taking great care to avoid damage to the sciatic nerve.

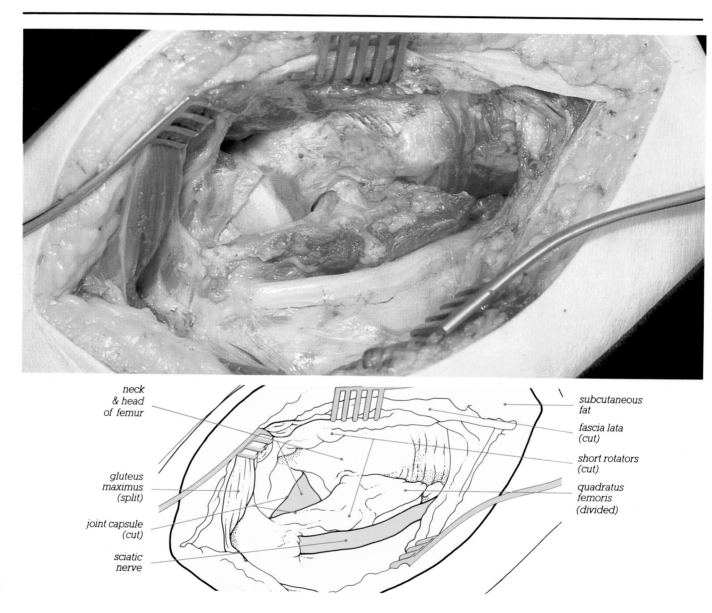

neck
& head
of femur

subcutaneous
fat

fascia lata
(cut)

short rotators
(cut)

gluteus
maximus
(split)

quadratus
femoris
(divided)

joint capsule
(cut)

sciatic
nerve

Fig. 25.5 The femoral head can now be dislocated posteriorly.

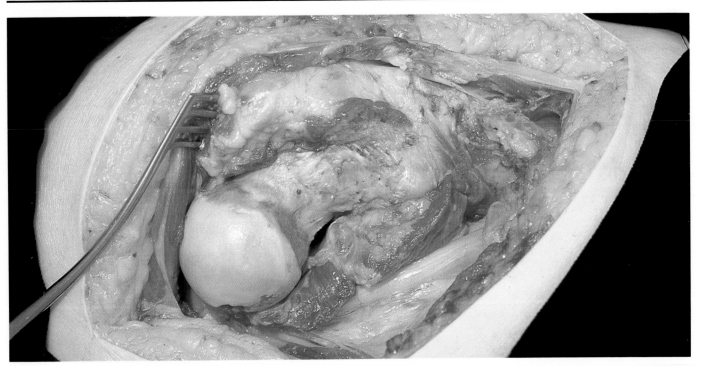

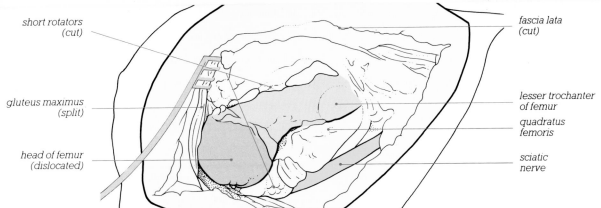

short rotators
(cut)

fascia lata
(cut)

gluteus maximus
(split)

lesser trochanter
of femur

quadratus
femoris

head of femur
(dislocated)

sciatic
nerve

2.17

26 Exposure of the Saphenofemoral Junction (Right)

Fig. 26.1 The incision is made 1cm below and parallel to the inguinal skin crease, centred just medial to the femoral pulse.

Points to consider

- There are usually five tributaries to the long saphenous vein at this junction, but the anatomy is variable.

- If performing a Trendelenburg procedure, ensure that no tributaries enter the saphenofemoral junction beneath the flush ligature.

- Take great care not to damage the femoral vein.

- The small superficial external pudendal artery is an almost constant finding. It may be advantageous to ligate and divide it to facilitate dissection of the saphenofemoral junction.

Position
The patient is supine with the leg slightly abducted, usually using the leg board across the end of the operating table. The table is tilted with the head downwards.

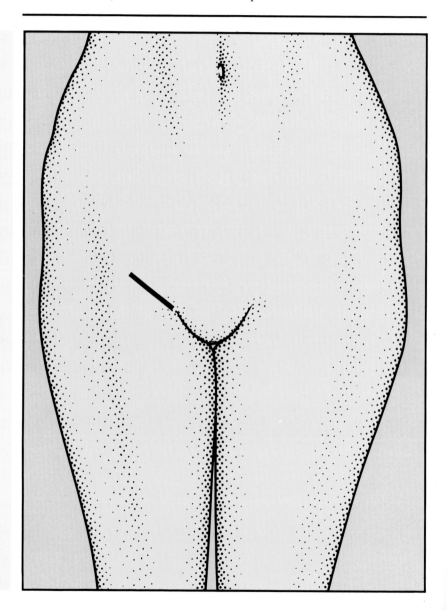

Fig. 26.2 The superficial fascia is carefully incised and the long saphenous vein and its tributaries identified. The tributaries are ligated and divided, and the long saphenous vein traced through the cribriform fascia to its junction with the femoral vein.

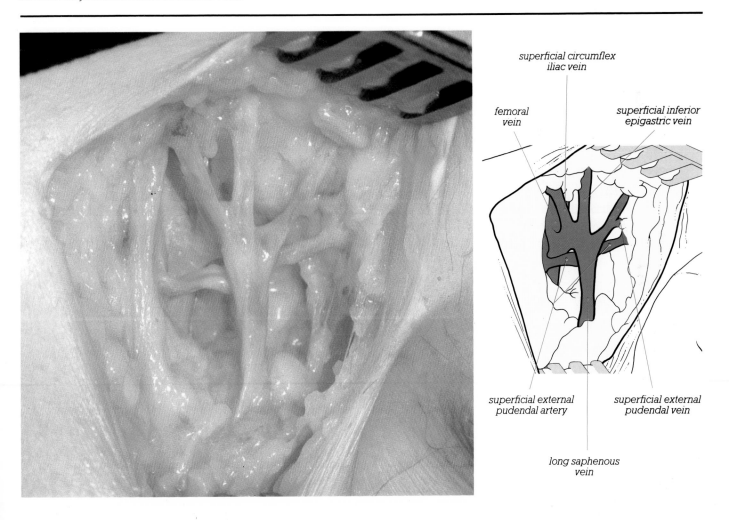

superficial circumflex
iliac vein

femoral
vein

superficial inferior
epigastric vein

superficial external
pudendal artery

superficial external
pudendal vein

long saphenous
vein

27 Exposure of the Common Femoral Artery and Origin of the Profunda Femoris Artery (Right)

Fig. 27.1 A 10cm vertical incision commences approximately 2.5cm proximal to the inguinal ligament and should lie over the femoral artery which, if not palpable, is identified at the midinguinal point.

Points to consider

- The profunda femoris artery occasionally arises as two vessels from the common femoral artery. Ensure that both are controlled before performing an arteriotomy.

- Always dissect adjacent to the arterial wall because the femoral nerve is immediately lateral and the femoral vein medial to the dissection (see Fig. 27.4).

- A transverse arteriotomy is preferred for embolectomy as there is no narrowing of the lumen when repaired.

Position

The patient is supine with both legs slightly abducted on a leg board. Both groins are prepared for an embolectomy. If done for a femoropopliteal bypass, the knee is flexed, the hip slightly externally rotated and the leg supported by sandbags beneath the knee and sole of the foot.

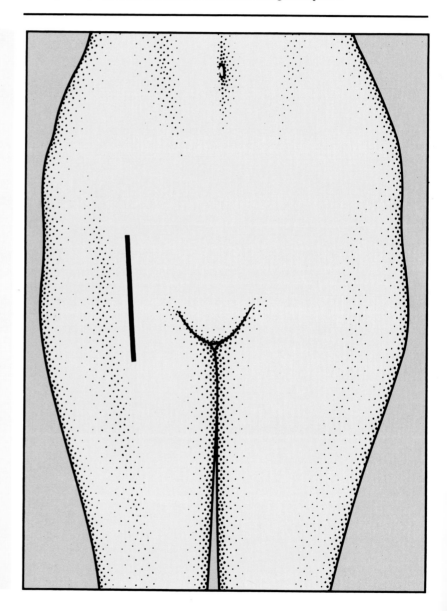

Fig. 27.2 The superficial fascia is incised and tributaries of the long saphenous vein ligated and divided as necessary (see Fig. 26.2). Even if there is no femoral pulse the femoral artery can often be felt as a solid 'finger' of tissue. The deep fascia is incised just lateral to the saphenofemoral junction to expose the artery.

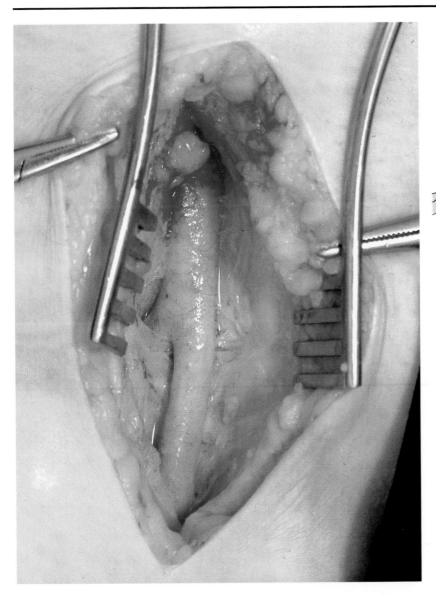

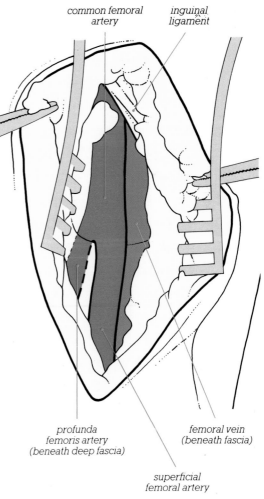

common femoral artery

inguinal ligament

profunda femoris artery (beneath deep fascia)

femoral vein (beneath fascia)

superficial femoral artery

2.21

Fig. 27.3 Keeping immediately adjacent to the arterial wall, the common and superficial femoral arteries are exposed circumferentially and slings passed around both. The length of artery exposed must be sufficient for easy application of an arterial clamp. Using the slings to apply traction to the femoral vessels, the profunda femoris artery is exposed and cleared circumferentially and a sling placed around this also.

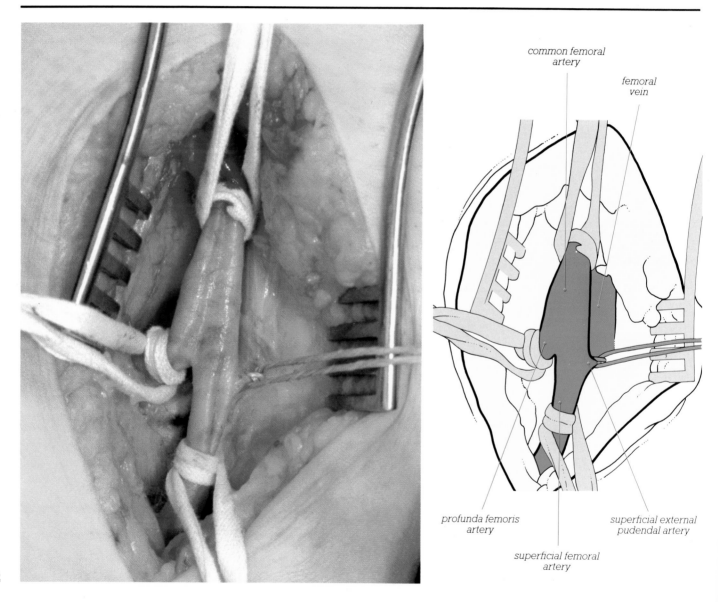

common femoral artery

femoral vein

profunda femoris artery

superficial external pudendal artery

superficial femoral artery

Fig. 27.4 Any smaller arterial branches should be controlled with silk or cotton ligatures passed around each vessel twice. If necessary for adequate exposure and control, these branches may be divided; but this is best avoided in the critically ischaemic limb. This extended exposure shows vulnerable structures.

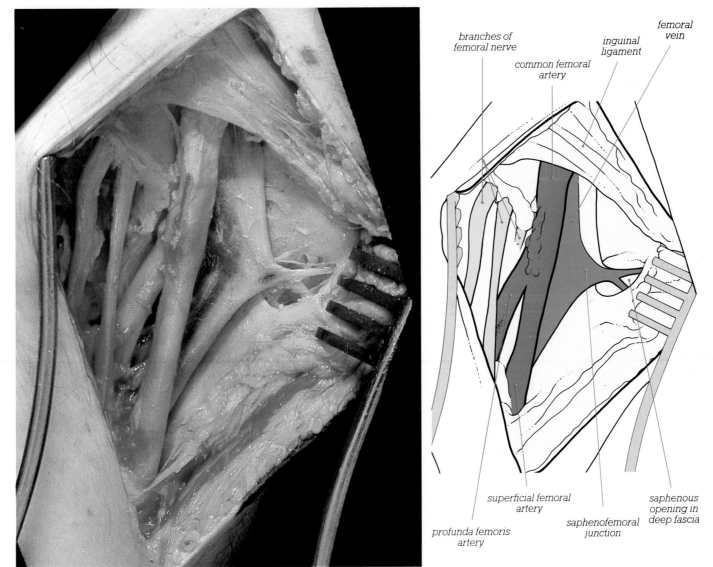

branches of femoral nerve

common femoral artery

inguinal ligament

femoral vein

superficial femoral artery

saphenofemoral junction

saphenous opening in deep fascia

profunda femoris artery

28 Block Dissection of the Groin (Right)

Fig. 28.1 The incision runs parallel to and 3cm below the inguinal ligament and may be extended distally by curving the incision over the medial side of the thigh.

Points to consider

- If the skin is obviously involved in the disease, it should be excised as an ellipse and removed *en bloc* with the superficial tissues.

- If necessary, iliac node dissection may be carried out in continuity by performing a retroperitoneal dissection above the inguinal ligament. This involves either dividing the inguinal ligament or making an incision through the anterior abdominal wall above the inguinal ligament. (A detailed description is outside the scope of this text but is well described in most standard surgical texts.)

Position
The patient is supine with the leg slightly abducted and the thigh externally rotated.

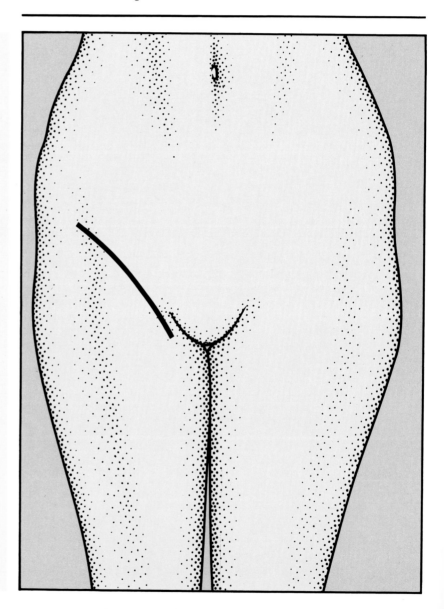

Fig. 28.2 An upper skin flap is raised to approximately 3cm above the inguinal ligament. At this level the superficial fascia is incised down to the external oblique aponeurosis along the length of the incision. The exposed layer of fatty tissue is dissected from the external oblique aponeurosis and reflected distally to the level of the inguinal ligament. A lower skin flap extends from the lateral edge of sartorius to the medial side of adductor longus, meeting the upper flap at the apex of the femoral triangle.

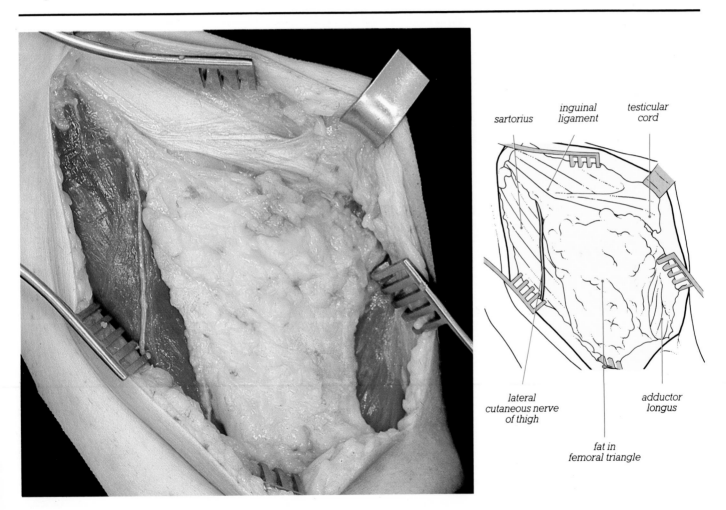

BLOCK DISSECTION OF THE GROIN (RIGHT)

Fig. 28.3 At the lateral edge of sàrtorius the superficial fascia, followed by the fascia lata, are incised and all tissue cleared medially from sartorius. The lateral and intermediate cutaneous nerves of the thigh should be found and preserved if possible. The femoral triangle is entered as dissection proceeds medially and the femoral nerve, artery and vein exposed and preserved. Superficial branches of the femoral artery are ligated and divided.

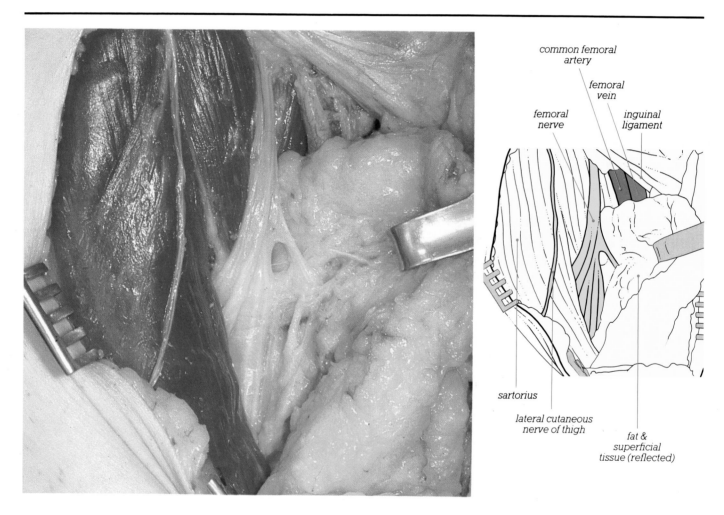

Fig. 28.4 At the saphenofemoral junction the long saphenous vein is identified and a flush ligation performed. The vein is then divided where it leaves the femoral triangle distally. The block of tissue is now cleared from adductor longus and deep fascia incised longitudinally over this muscle. In the femoral canal, the tissue remains attached to lymphatics which are drawn down for removal of the lymph nodes, completing the dissection.

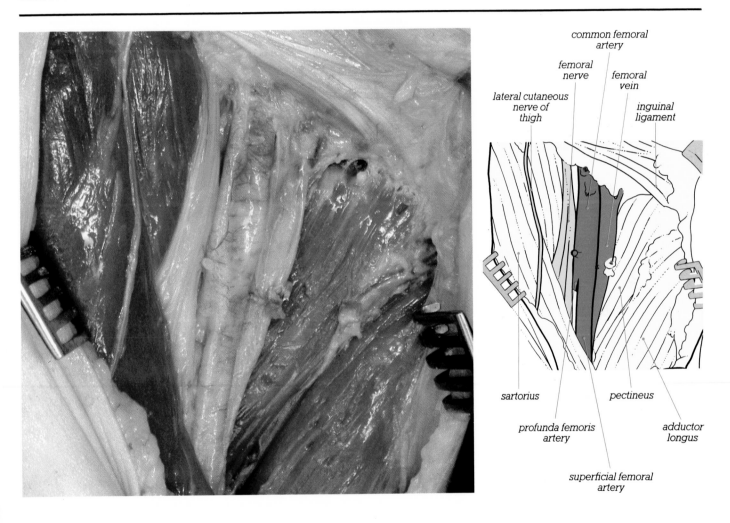

common femoral artery

femoral nerve

femoral vein

lateral cutaneous nerve of thigh

inguinal ligament

sartorius

pectineus

profunda femoris artery

adductor longus

superficial femoral artery

29 Posterolateral Approach to the Femur (Left)

Fig. 29.1 The incision is made over the posterolateral surface of the femur.

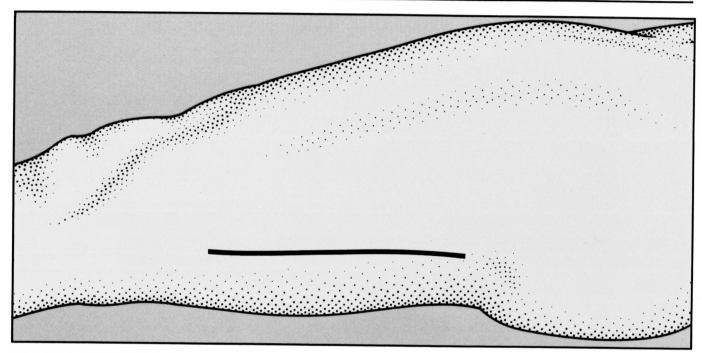

Points to consider
- This is a safe exposure as the quadriceps muscle is retracted rather than cut and the sciatic nerve is protected by the lateral intermuscular septum.

Position
The patient is placed on the sound side, supported by anterior and posterior cushions. Draping allows free movement of the affected hip and knee.

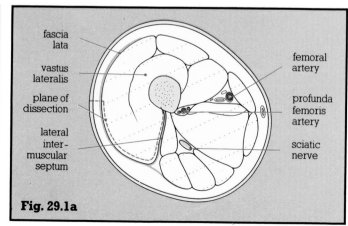

fascia lata

vastus lateralis

plane of dissection

lateral inter-muscular septum

femoral artery

profunda femoris artery

sciatic nerve

Fig. 29.1a

Fig. 29.2 The incision is deepened to expose the fascia lata.

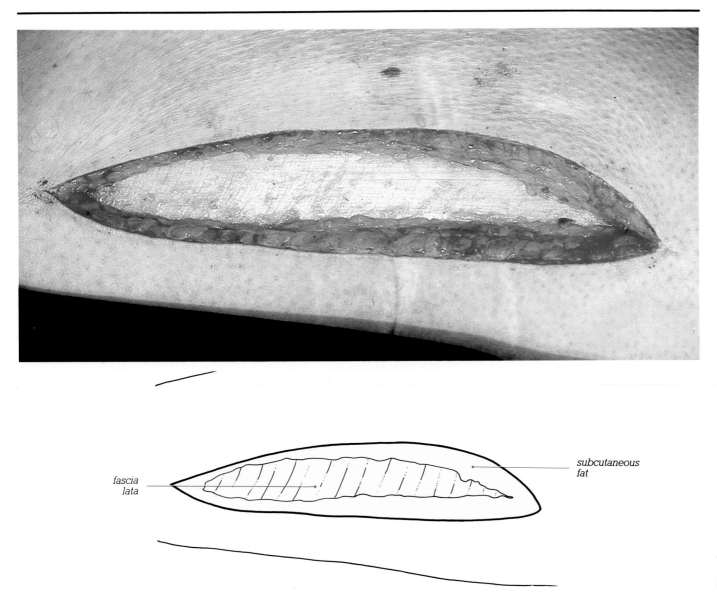

fascia lata

subcutaneous fat

Fig. 29.3 The fascia lata is split in the same line as the skin incision to expose vastus lateralis.

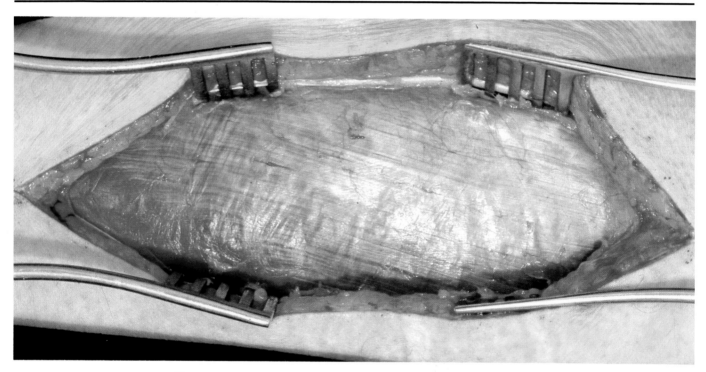

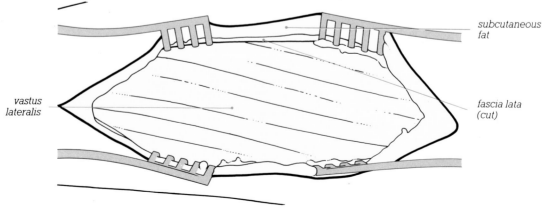

subcutaneous
fat

vastus
lateralis

fascia lata
(cut)

Fig. 29.4 A plane is developed posteriorly between vastus lateralis and the lateral intermuscular septum. Vastus lateralis is then retracted anteriorly and perforating vessels from the profunda femoris artery identified and ligated.

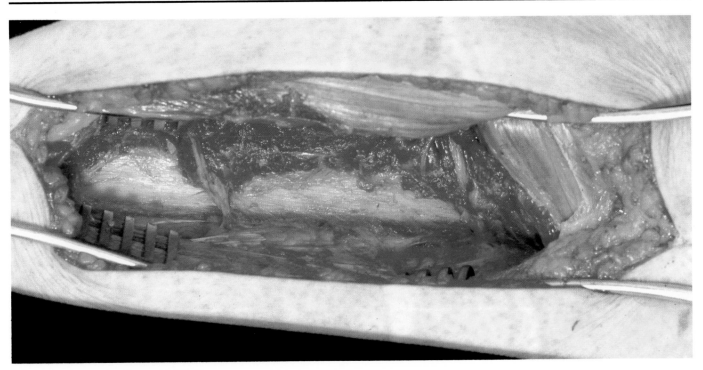

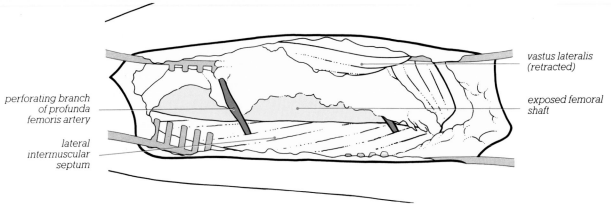

vastus lateralis
(retracted)

perforating branch
of profunda
femoris artery

exposed femoral
shaft

lateral
intermuscular
septum

2.31

Fig. 29.5 Further dissection allows a good exposure of the femoral shaft.

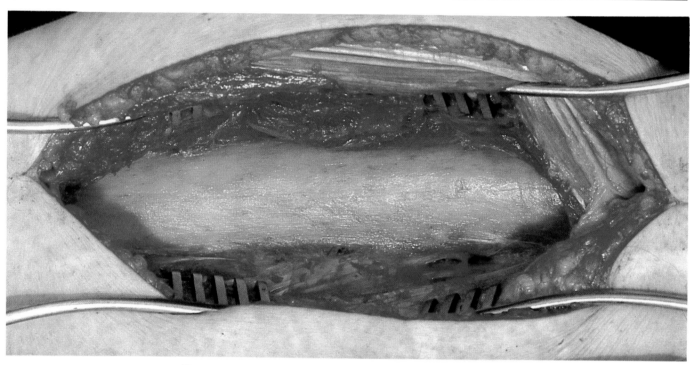

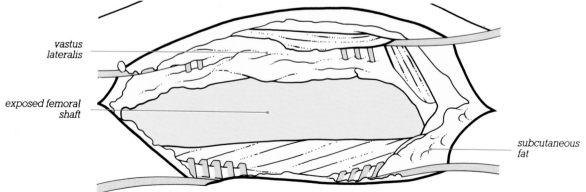

vastus
lateralis

exposed femoral
shaft

subcutaneous
fat

Approach to the Supracondylar Region of the Femur (Left)

Fig. 30.1 The incision runs along the lateral aspect of the femur, just in front of the iliotibial tract, from a point 10-15cm proximal to the joint line. Distally the incision is curved forwards towards the tibial tubercle.

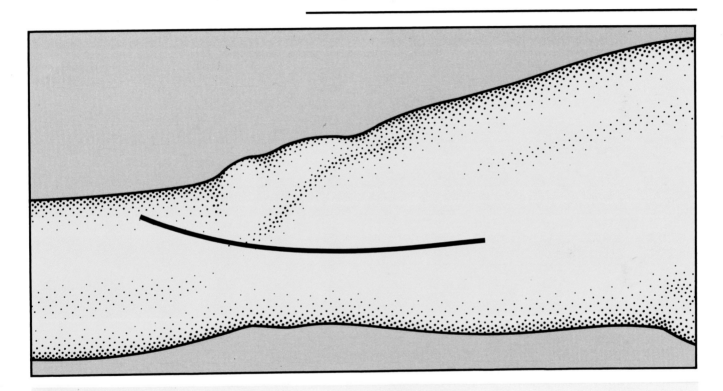

Points to consider

- The sciatic nerve is protected by an intact lateral intermuscular septum.

Position

The patient is supine with the leg straight, a sandbag under the ipsilateral buttock and a tourniquet around the most proximal part of the thigh.

Fig. 30.2 The fascia lata is exposed, then incised along the same line.

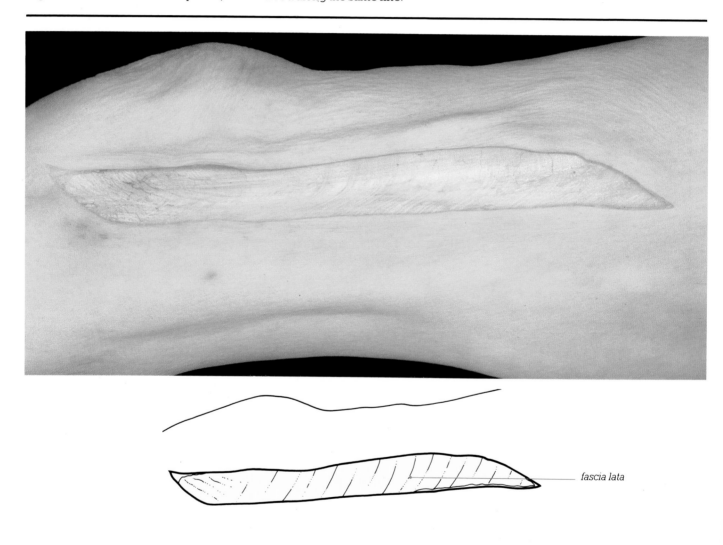

fascia lata

Fig. 30.3 Vastus lateralis is lifted away anteriorly from the intermuscular septum, and perforating branches of the profunda femoris artery are identified and divided.

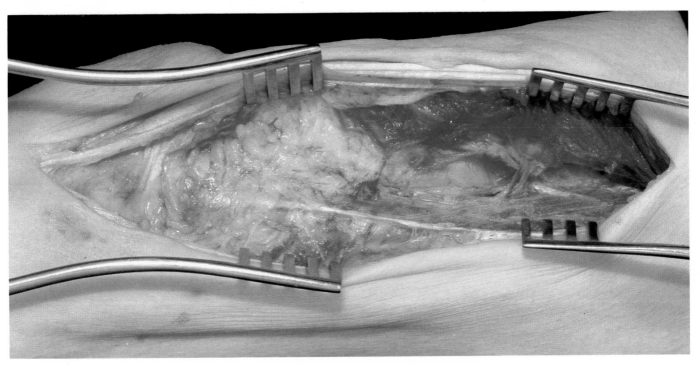

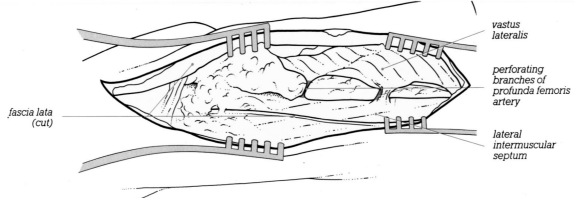

vastus
lateralis

perforating
branches of
profunda femoris
artery

lateral
intermuscular
septum

fascia lata
(cut)

2.35

Fig. 30.4 Vastus lateralis is separated from its attachment to the linea aspera, exposing the supracondylar region of the femoral shaft.

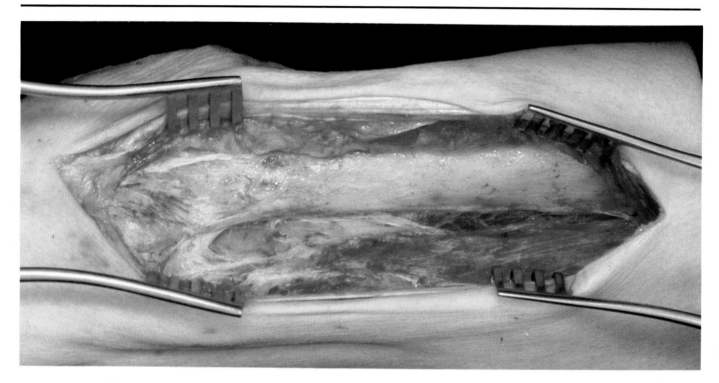

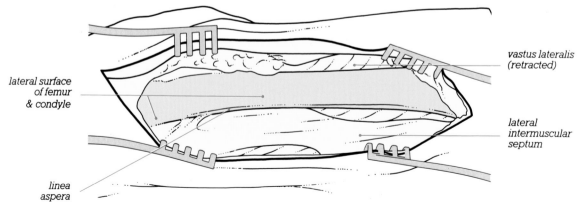

lateral surface
of femur
& condyle

vastus lateralis
(retracted)

lateral
intermuscular
septum

linea
aspera

Fig. 30.5 To obtain better exposure distally, the joint capsule is divided in the same line as the skin incision and the extensor apparatus retracted medially.

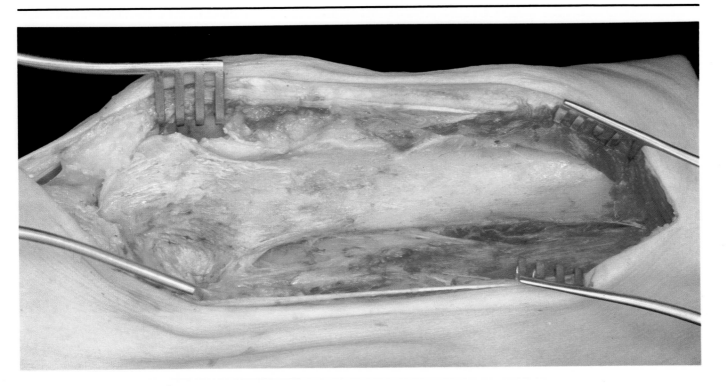

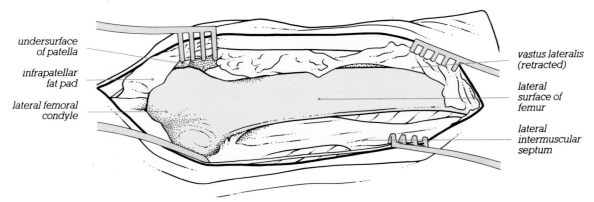

undersurface of patella

infrapatellar fat pad

lateral femoral condyle

vastus lateralis (retracted)

lateral surface of femur

lateral intermuscular septum

2.37

31 Exposure of the Proximal Popliteal Artery (Right)

Fig. 31.1 The incision runs longitudinally along the medial aspect of the lower third of the thigh, centred on the adductor tubercle, along a line drawn from the midinguinal point to the adductor tubercle.

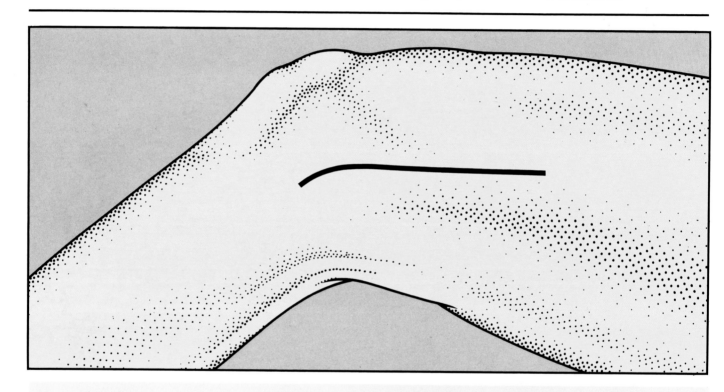

Points to consider

- The tendon of adductor magnus may be divided to increase exposure, but ensure that adequate tendon remains distally for repair at the end of the operation.

- A transverse arteriotomy is made if performing an embolectomy as there is no narrowing of the lumen when repaired.

Position

The patient is supine with the hip and knee flexed and the thigh externally rotated. The leg is supported by sandbags.

Fig. 31.2 The superficial and deep fascia are incised anterior to sartorius and the latter retracted posteriorly. Dissection is carried on beneath vastus medialis to identify the tendon of adductor magnus.

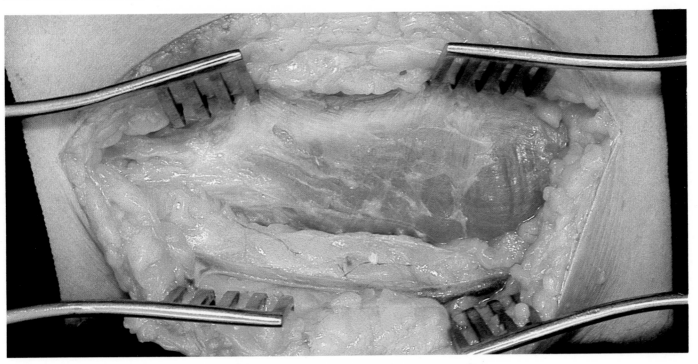

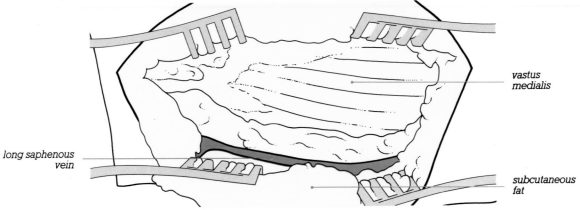

vastus medialis

long saphenous vein

subcutaneous fat

2.39

Fig. 31.3 The fascia is incised immediately posterior to the adductor tendon, entering the fatty tissue of the popliteal fossa. Using blunt dissection in the fat the popliteal vessels are identified, the artery being adjacent to the femur at this level.

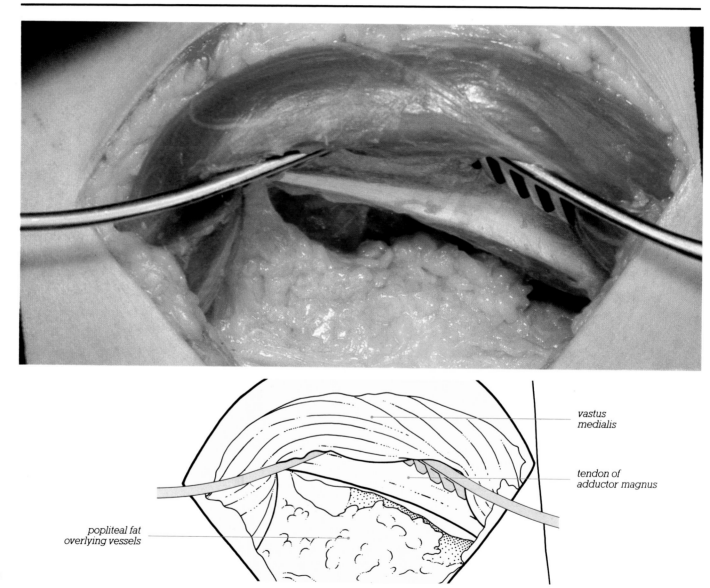

vastus
medialis

tendon of
adductor magnus

popliteal fat
overlying vessels

Fig. 31.4 Dissecting close to the arterial wall the artery is cleared circumferentially and slings placed around it proximally and distally. Any geniculate branches should be controlled with silk slings.

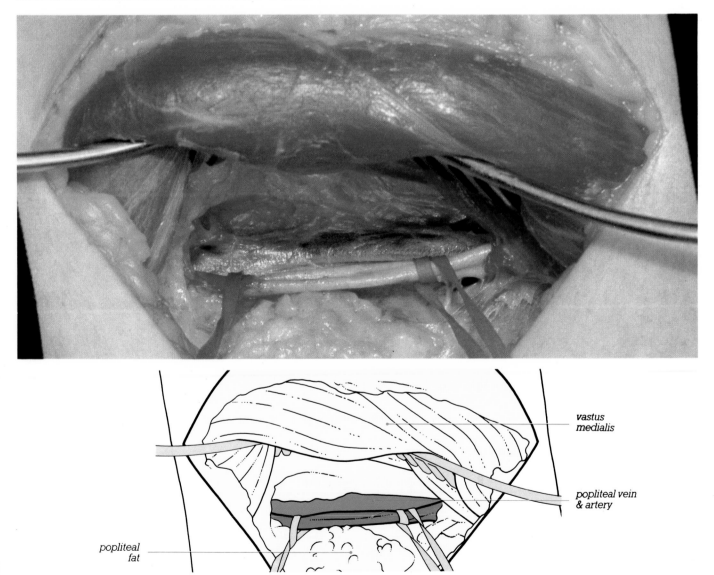

vastus medialis

popliteal vein & artery

popliteal fat

32 Transverse Anterior Approach to the Knee Joint (Right)

Fig. 32.1 The incision is 2mm below the tibial plateau and extends over the medial and lateral collateral ligaments of the knee.

Points to consider

- A bone lever inserted through the intercondylar notch of the femur to push the tibia forward will protect the neurovascular structures in the popliteal fossa.

- This incision destroys the integrity of the joint and is used only for arthrodesis or total arthroplasty.

Position
The patient is supine with the hip flexed and the knee flexed to one hundred and twenty degrees. A tourniquet may or may not be used.

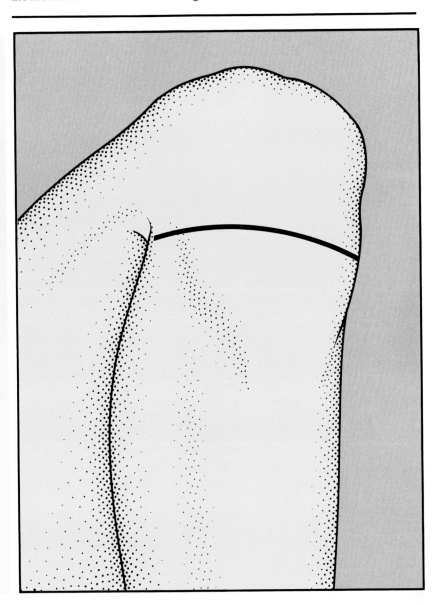

Fig. 32.2 The incision is deepened as far as the joint capsule.

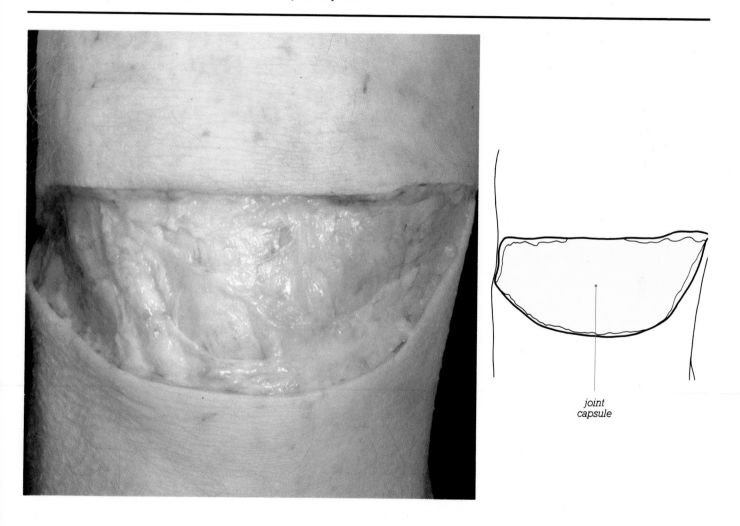

joint
capsule

Fig. 32.3 The capsule is opened in the same line as the incision by incising the patellar ligament and its expansions.

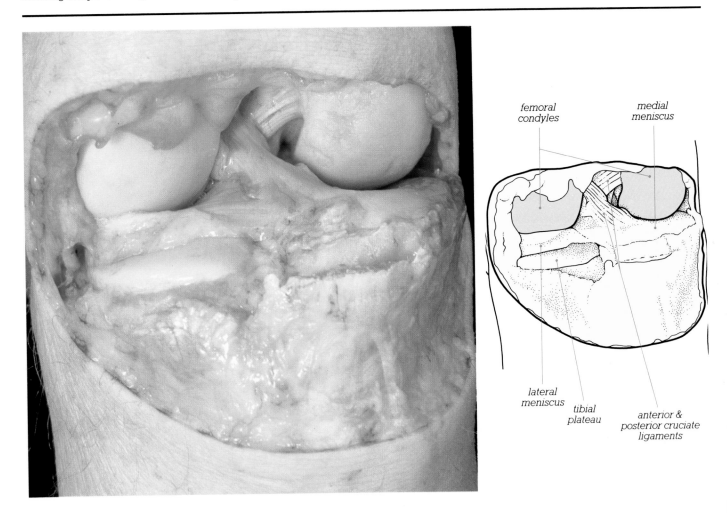

femoral condyles

medial meniscus

lateral meniscus

tibial plateau

anterior & posterior cruciate ligaments

Fig. 32.4 The medial and lateral collateral ligaments and the anterior cruciate ligament have been divided and both menisci removed.

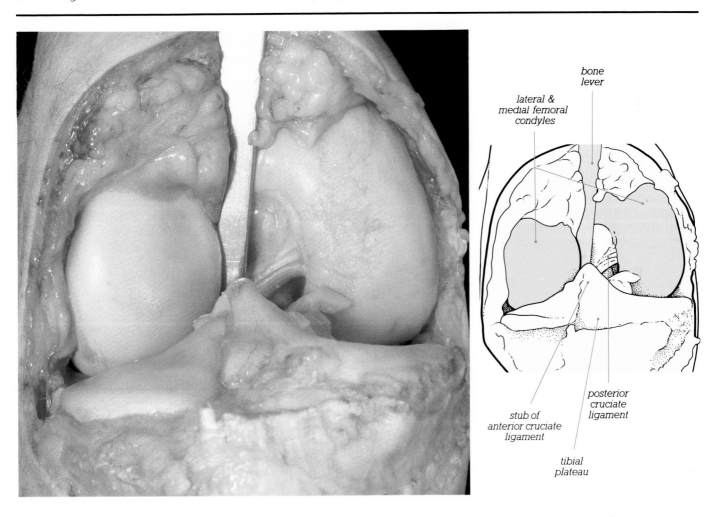

bone
lever

lateral &
medial femoral
condyles

posterior
cruciate
ligament

stub of
anterior cruciate
ligament

tibial
plateau

33 Anteromedial Approach to the Knee Joint (Right)

Fig. 33.1 The incision skirts the medial border of the patella and continues longitudinally over the tibial condyle and along the medial border of the tendon of rectus femoris proximally.

Points to consider

- The infrapatellar branch of the saphenous nerve should be identified in the distal part of the incision and, if possible, preserved.

- A sufficient cuff of tissue should be left on the medial border of the patella to allow adequate reattachment. At the end of the procedure, ensure normal tracking of the patella.

Position
The patient is supine with the knee extended and a tourniquet around the upper thigh. The leg is draped to allow free movement.

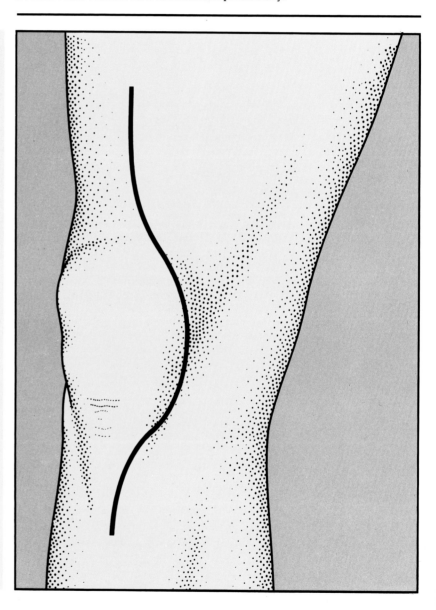

Fig. 33.2 The incision is deepened to expose the fibrous capsule of the knee joint.

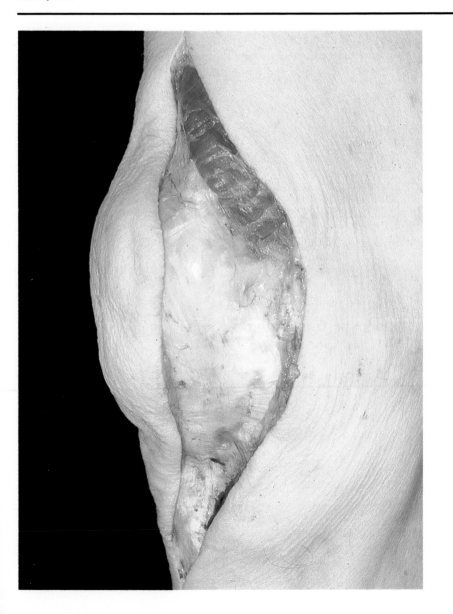

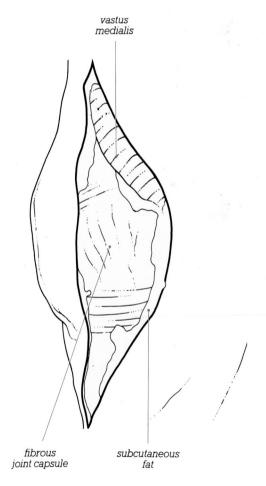

vastus medialis

fibrous joint capsule

subcutaneous fat

2.47

Fig. 33.3 Vastus medialis is detached from its insertion to the quadriceps tendon and the joint opened in the same line as the skin incision.

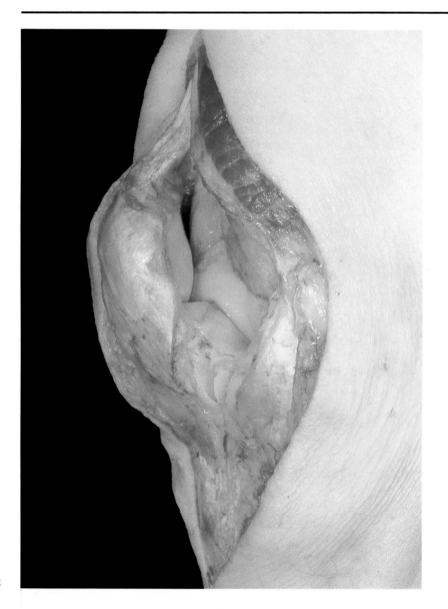

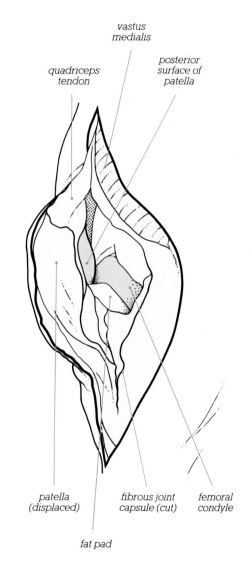

vastus
medialis

quadriceps
tendon

posterior
surface of
patella

patella
(displaced)

fibrous joint
capsule (cut)

femoral
condyle

fat pad

Fig. 33.4 Flexion of the knee and lateral dislocation of the patella allow good exposure of anterior intra-articular structures.

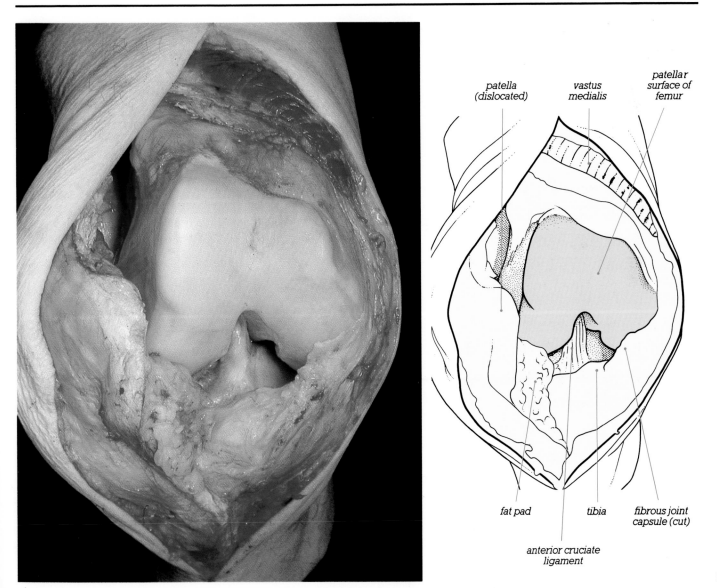

patella (dislocated)

vastus medialis

patellar surface of femur

fat pad

tibia

fibrous joint capsule (cut)

anterior cruciate ligament

2.49

34 Parapatellar Approach to the Medial Meniscus (Left)

Fig. 34.1 The 2cm incision runs medial to the medial edge of the patella, just overlapping the upper edge of the tibial plateau.

Points to consider

- The infrapatellar branch of the saphenous nerve, which runs laterally across the medial tibial condyle to supply cutaneous sensation below the patella, has a variable course and may be damaged particularly if the incision is extended distally.

- If problems arise when removing the posterior horn of the medial meniscus, a posteromedial incision may be useful (see Figs. 35.1-35.4).

Position

The patient is supine with the knee flexed over the end of the table. A tourniquet is around the upper thigh and a sandbag is under the thigh.

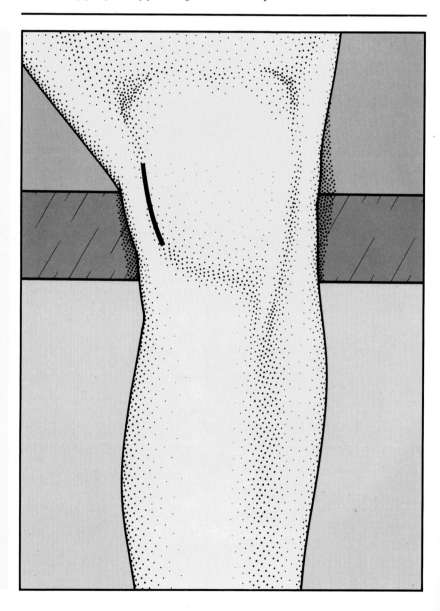

Fig. 34.2 The fibrous capsule of the knee joint is incised in the same line as the skin incision.

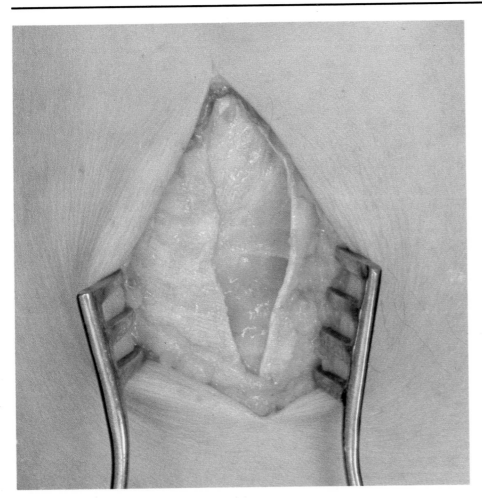

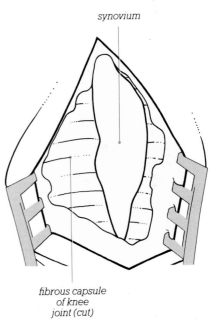

synovium

fibrous capsule
of knee
joint (cut)

Fig. 34.3 The synovial membrane is incised in the same line as the skin incision. A blunt hook has been inserted around the anterior horn of the medial meniscus.

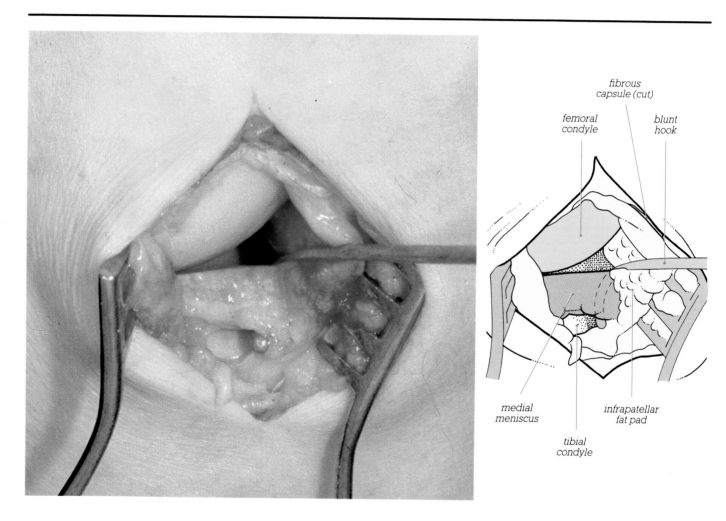

fibrous
capsule (cut)

femoral
condyle

blunt
hook

medial
meniscus

infrapatellar
fat pad

tibial
condyle

Fig. 34.4 The incision has been extended to show associated structures
of the medial meniscus and allow improved access.

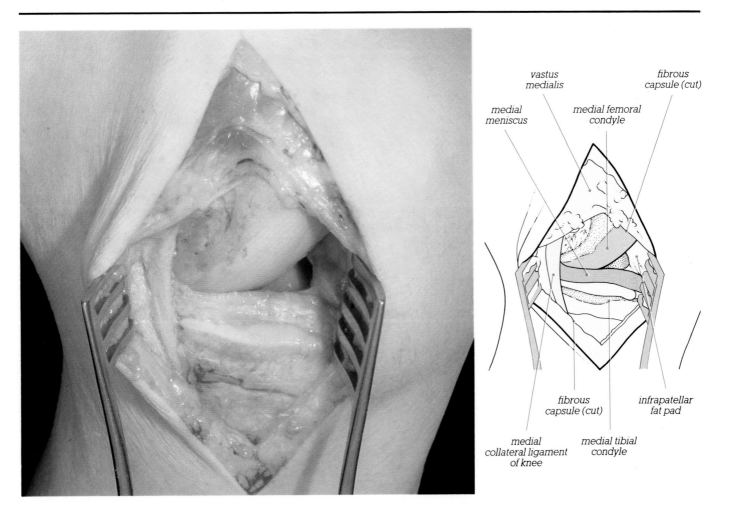

vastus
medialis

fibrous
capsule (cut)

medial
meniscus

medial femoral
condyle

fibrous
capsule (cut)

infrapatellar
fat pad

medial
collateral ligament
of knee

medial tibial
condyle

35 Posteromedial Approach to the Knee Joint (Right)

Fig. 35.1 The longitudinal incision starts behind the medial collateral ligament of the knee and runs across the medial femoral condyle to the tibial plateau.

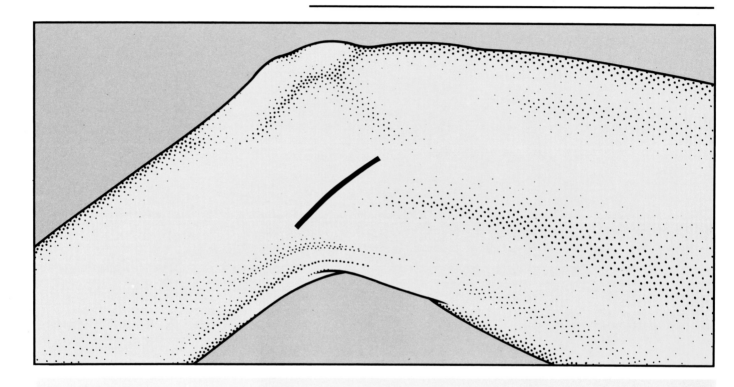

Points to consider

- This is usually a second incision for removal of the posterior horn of a medial meniscus which has not been achieved using the medial parapatellar approach (see Figs. 34.1-34.4).

- A pair of blunt forceps inside the knee will allow the posterior border of the medial collateral ligament to be clearly defined and preserved.

Position
The patient is supine with the hip flexed, abducted and externally rotated to allow full flexion of the knee. A tourniquet is placed around the thigh.

Fig. 35.2 The capsule is opened by deepening the incision and incising the oblique fibres of the posterior part of the medial collateral ligament, taking care to preserve the longitudinal fibres.

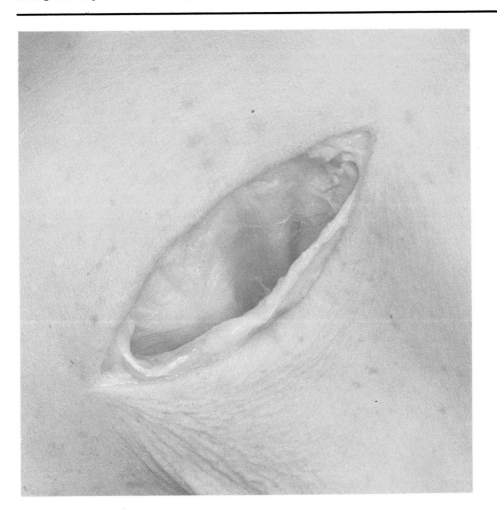

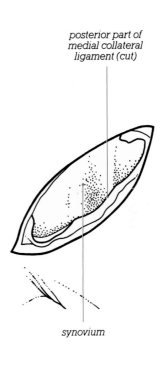

posterior part of medial collateral ligament (cut)

synovium

Fig. 35.3 Retraction of the medial collateral ligament anteriorly and the hamstrings posteriorly gives a good view of the posterior horn of the medial meniscus.

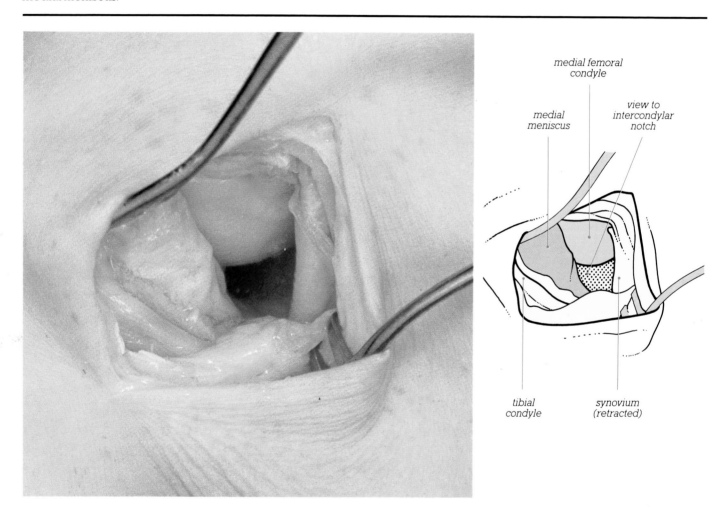

medial femoral condyle

medial meniscus

view to intercondylar notch

tibial condyle

synovium (retracted)

Fig. 35.4 An extended dissection demonstrates the adjacent structures.
This degree of exposure is seldom necessary.

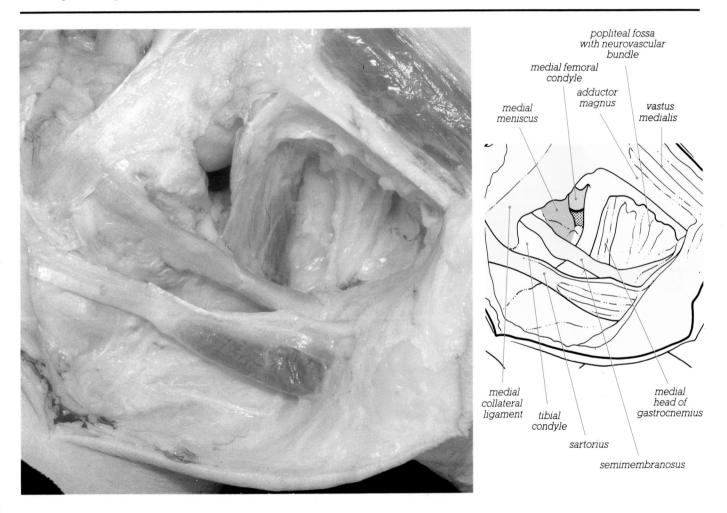

poplliteal fossa
with neurovascular
bundle

medial femoral
condyle

adductor
magnus

medial
meniscus

vastus
medialis

medial
collateral
ligament

tibial
condyle

sartorius

medial
head of
gastrocnemius

semimembranosus

36 Approach to the Lateral Meniscus (Right)

Fig. 36.1 The transverse incision is made 2mm below the joint line and runs from the lateral edge of the patellar ligament to the anterior edge of the lateral collateral ligament.

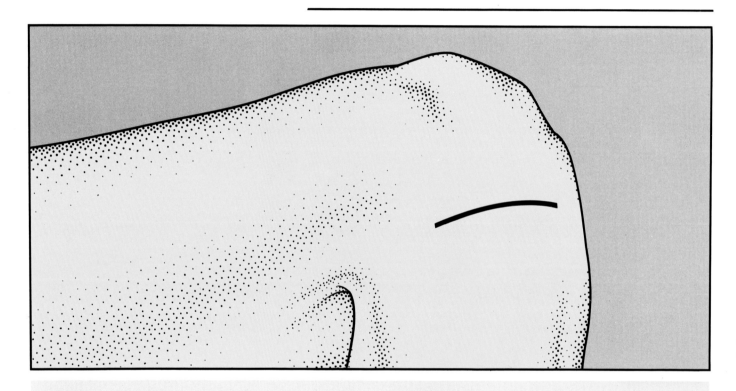

Points to consider
- The lateral inferior geniculate artery runs round the rim of the lateral meniscus between the lateral collateral ligament and synovium.

- If there is difficulty in removing the posterior horn of the meniscus, the posterolateral approach may be helpful (see Figs. 37.1-37.5).

Position
The patient is supine with the hip flexed to allow full flexion of the knee. A tourniquet is placed around the thigh.

Fig. 36.2 The incision is deepened to expose the iliotibial tract.

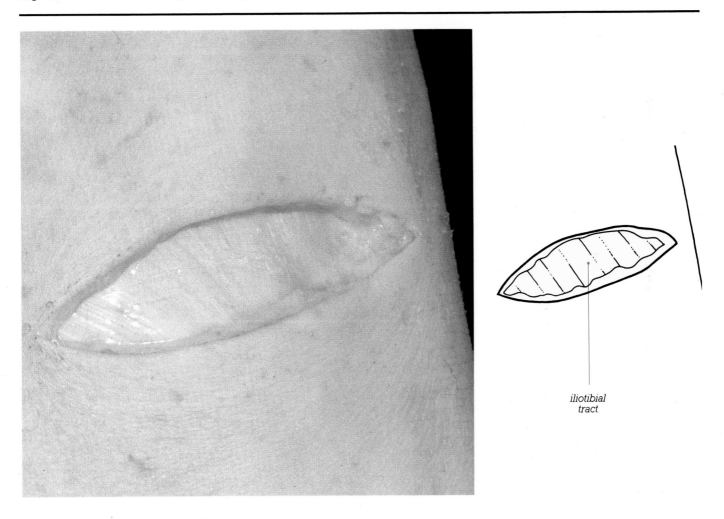

iliotibial
tract

Fig. 36.3 Incision of the iliotibial tract in the direction of its fibres exposes the lateral meniscus.

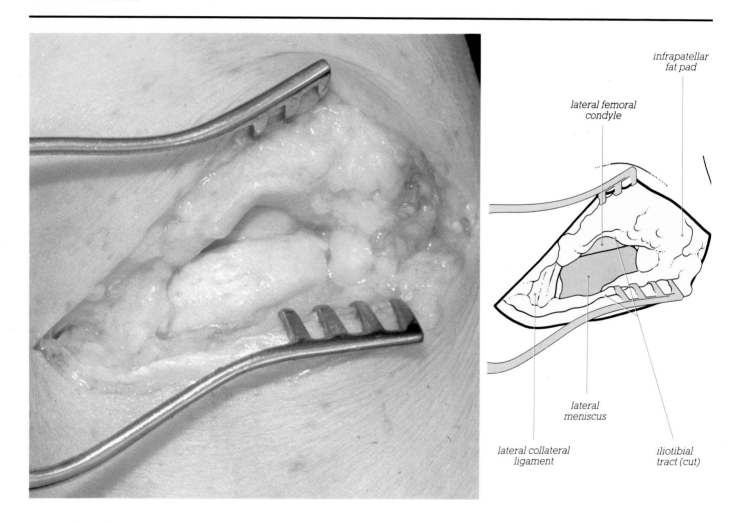

infrapatellar
fat pad

lateral femoral
condyle

lateral
meniscus

lateral collateral
ligament

iliotibial
tract (cut)

Posterolateral Approach to the Knee Joint (Right)

Fig. 37.1 The incision runs along the posterior border of the iliotibial tract, then curves across the head of the fibula.

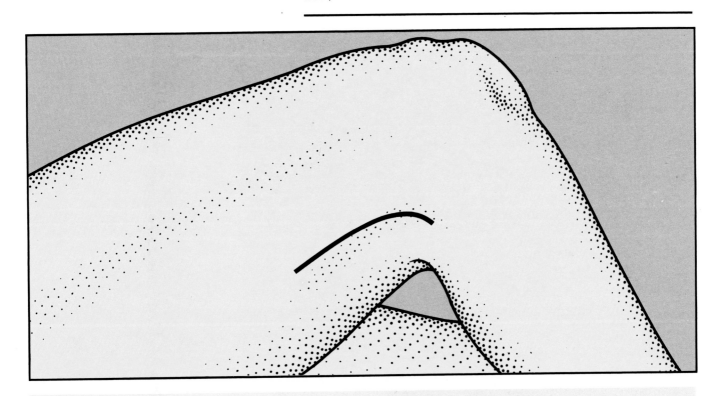

Points to consider

- At the level of this approach, popliteus is intracapsular and may have to be retracted laterally.

- This approach is commonly used for removal of the posterior horn of the lateral meniscus if it cannot be removed using the anterior approach (see Figs. 36.1-36.3).

Position

The patient is supine and the hip flexed, allowing flexion of the knee. A tourniquet is placed around the thigh.

Fig. 37.2 The posterior border of the fascia lata is split from the deep fascia to reveal biceps femoris.

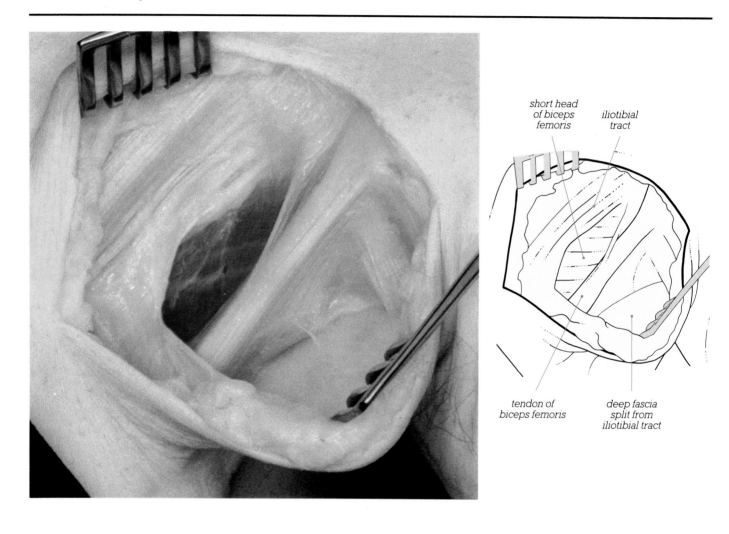

short head
of biceps
femoris

iliotibial
tract

tendon of
biceps femoris

deep fascia
split from
iliotibial tract

Fig. 37.3 The joint capsule is exposed between the fascia lata and the tendon of biceps femoris.

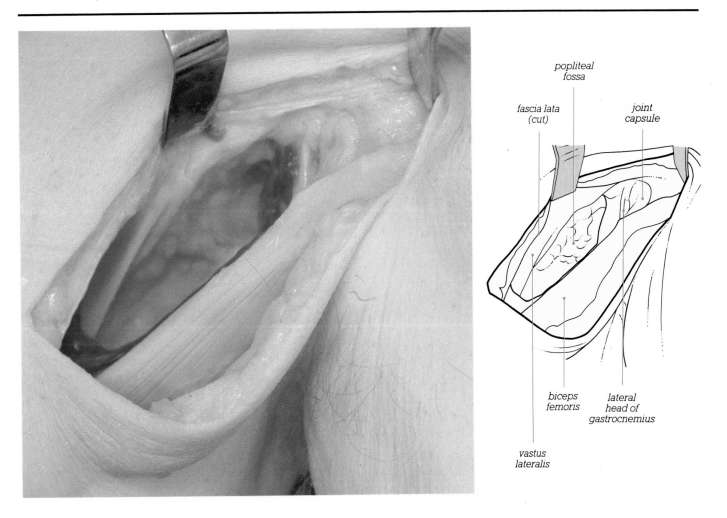

popliteal
fossa

fascia lata
(cut)

joint
capsule

biceps
femoris

lateral
head of
gastrocnemius

vastus
lateralis

Fig. 37.4 The joint capsule is incised, having retracted the lateral head of gastrocnemius posteriorly.

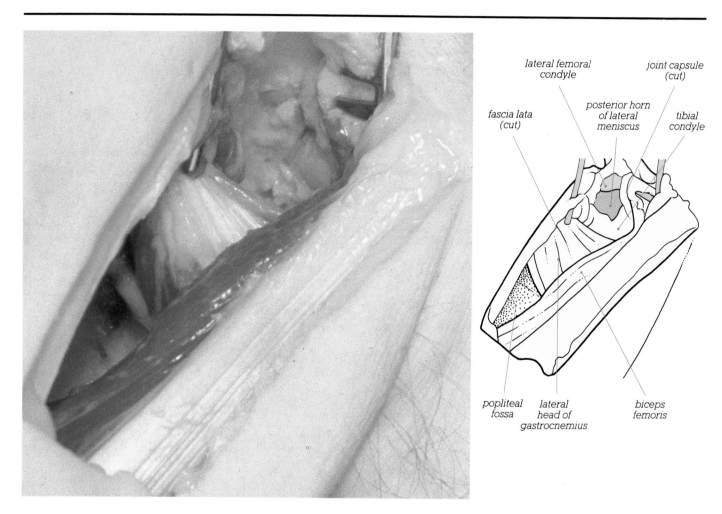

lateral femoral
condyle

joint capsule
(cut)

fascia lata
(cut)

posterior horn
of lateral
meniscus

tibial
condyle

popliteal
fossa

lateral
head of
gastrocnemius

biceps
femoris

Fig. 37.5 An extended dissection demonstrates the proximity of the common peroneal nerve and the popliteal neurovascular bundle. This degree of dissection is never necessary.

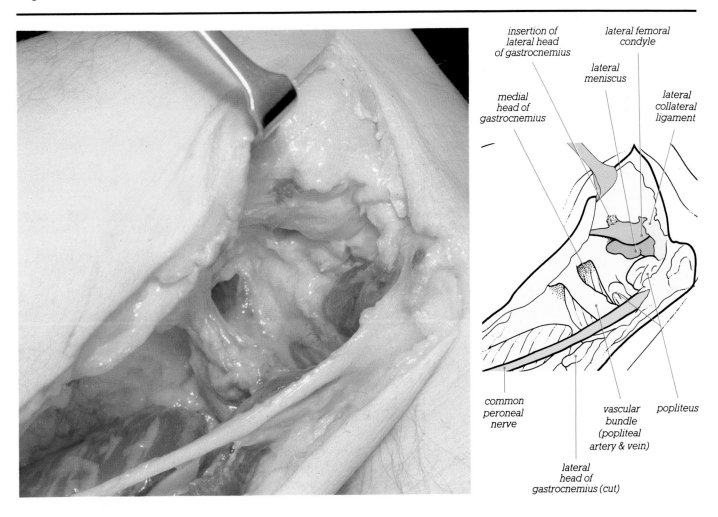

insertion of
lateral head
of gastrocnemius

lateral femoral
condyle

lateral
meniscus

medial
head of
gastrocnemius

lateral
collateral
ligament

common
peroneal
nerve

vascular
bundle
(popliteal
artery & vein)

popliteus

lateral
head of
gastrocnemius (cut)

38 Exposure of the Short Saphenopopliteal Venous Junction (Right)

Fig. 38.1 A sigmoid incision runs transversely in the popliteal skin crease at the level of the joint line and extends proximally on the lateral side of the thigh and distally on the medial side of the calf.

Points to consider

- The short saphenous vein frequently passes through the deep fascia at a variable distance below the popliteal fossa before running into the fossa itself. A wide exposure may be necessary for safe and effective exploration.

- There is often a posteromedial communicating branch between the long and short saphenous veins which leaves the short saphenous vein high up and passes medially into the thigh (see Fig. 38.2). This communicating branch should always be ligated and divided.

Position
The patient is prone with a small sandbag under the dorsum of the foot. No tourniquet is used.

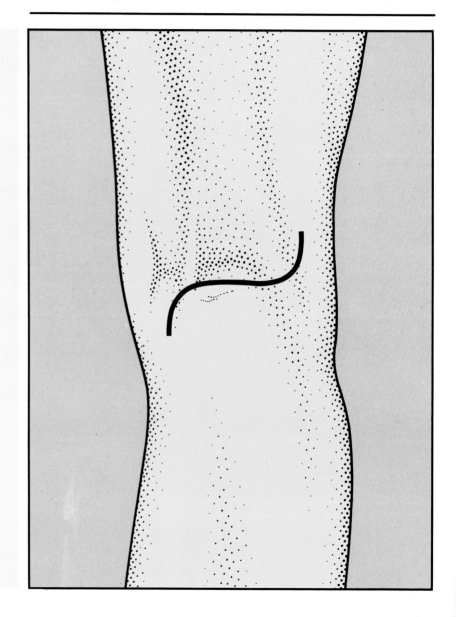

Fig. 38.2 The fascia is incised transversely and the short saphenous vein identified. Taking care not to damage the sural or tibial nerves, the short saphenous vein is followed down through the fat of the popliteal fossa to its junction with the popliteal vein. The popliteal artery lies deeper and need not be disturbed (see Figs. 40.1-40.5).

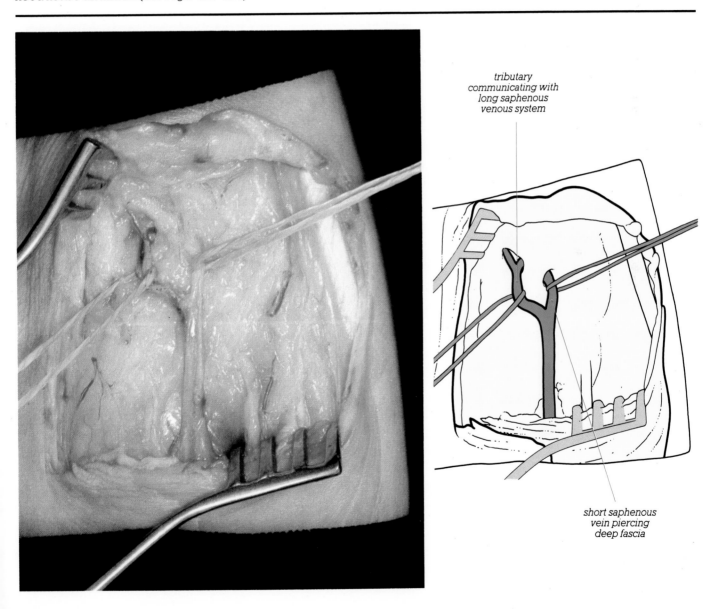

tributary
communicating with
long saphenous
venous system

short saphenous
vein piercing
deep fascia

2.67

Fig. 38.3 A flush ligation of the short saphenopopliteal junction is performed, if required.

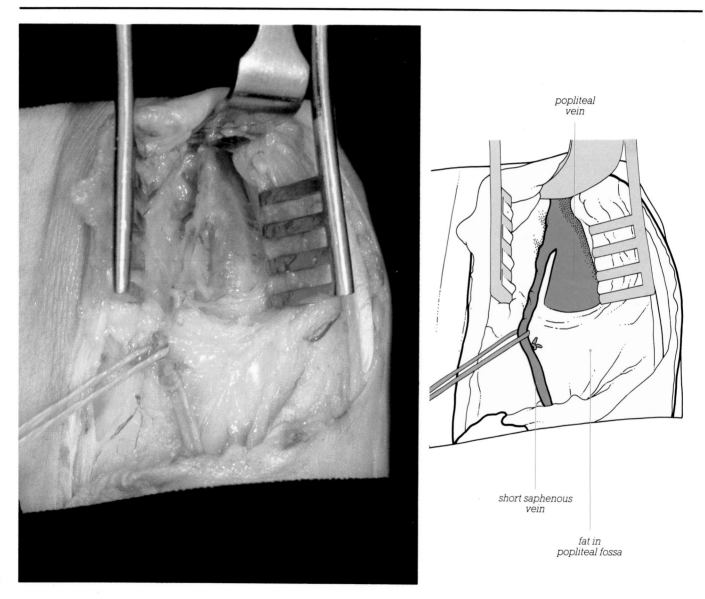

popliteal
vein

short saphenous
vein

fat in
popliteal fossa

Posterior Approach to the Popliteal Artery (Right)

Points to consider

- This is a good exposure for popliteal embolectomy.

- If arteriotomy is to be performed, a transverse one is preferred.

- In the popliteal fossa the common peroneal nerve receives a large vasa nervorum which, if damaged during operation, may result in a foot drop.

Position
The patient is prone with the knee extended over a small cushion under the patella.

Fig. 39.1 A sigmoid incision runs transversely in the popliteal skin crease and extends proximally on the medial side of the thigh and distally on the lateral side of the calf.

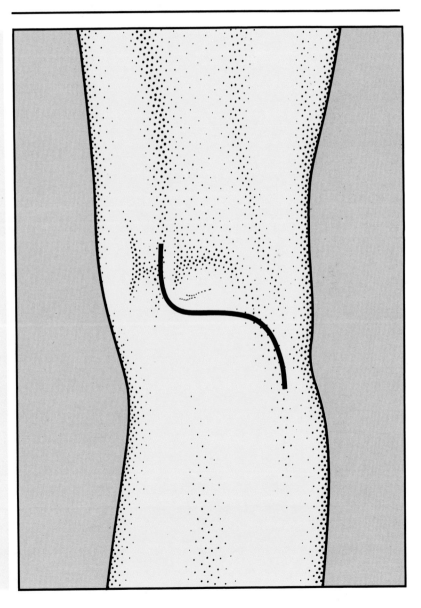

2.69

Fig. 39.2 The short saphenous vein, often lying deep to the deep fascia at this level, is identified.

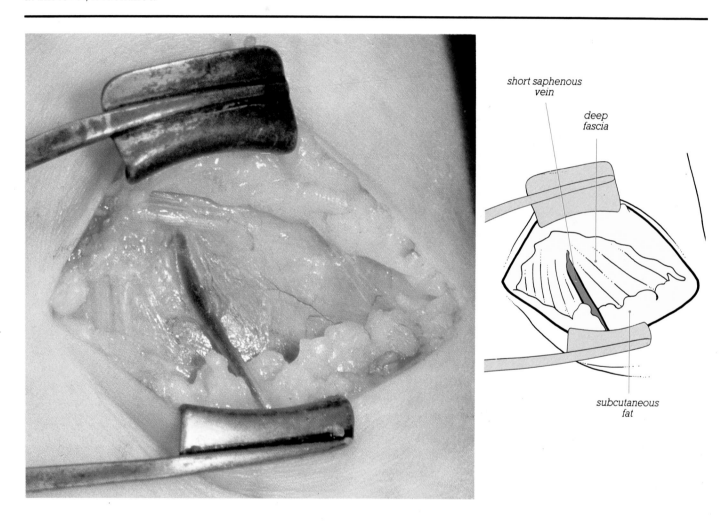

Fig. 39.3 The short saphenous vein is traced through the deep fascia to the popliteal vein.

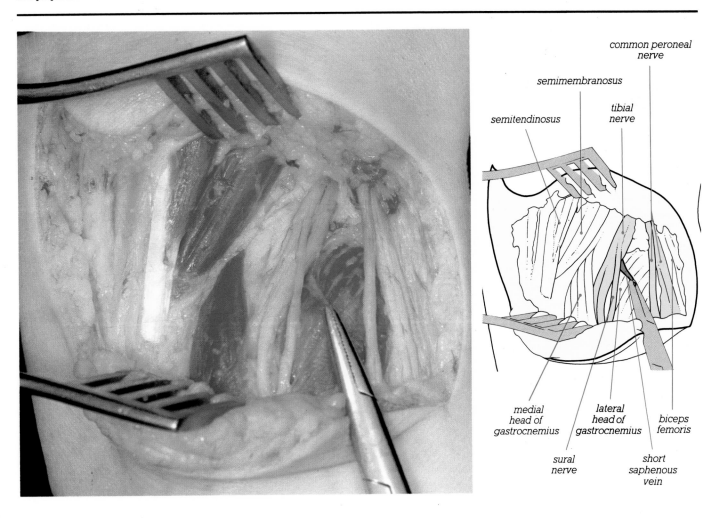

common peroneal
nerve

semimembranosus

tibial
nerve

semitendinosus

medial
head of
gastrocnemius

lateral
head of
gastrocnemius

biceps
femoris

sural
nerve

short
saphenous
vein

Fig. 39.4 The tibial and common peroneal nerves are preserved by gentle retraction and the popliteal vein dissected from the deeper popliteal artery. Once the artery is identified, all dissection should be carried out immediately adjacent to the arterial wall.

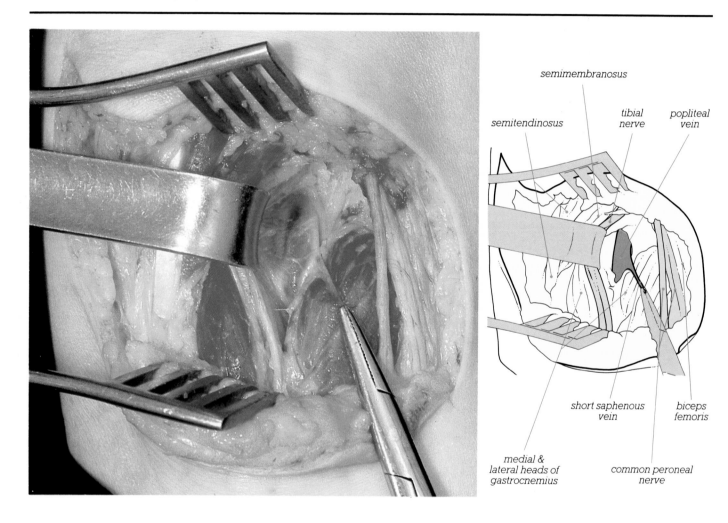

semimembranosus

semitendinosus

tibial nerve

popliteal vein

short saphenous vein

biceps femoris

medial & lateral heads of gastrocnemius

common peroneal nerve

Fig. 39.5 The popliteal artery is freed circumferentially as far proximally and distally as necessary for slings to be placed around the artery and any genicular branches.

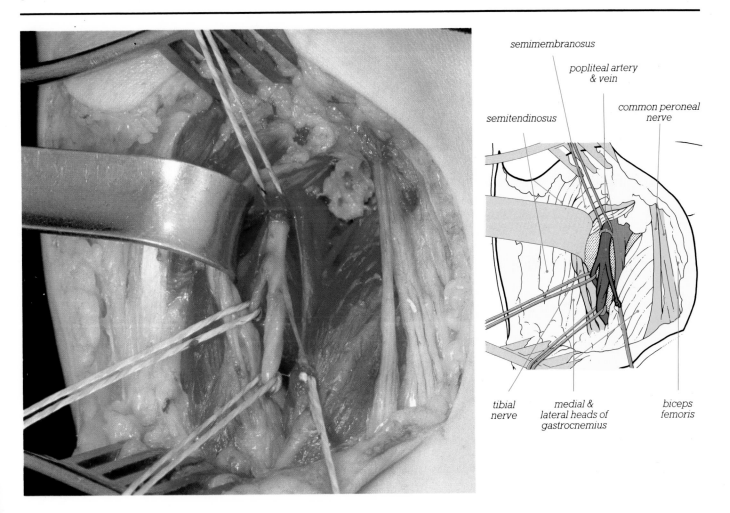

semimembranosus

popliteal artery
& vein

semitendinosus

common peroneal
nerve

tibial
nerve

medial &
lateral heads of
gastrocnemius

biceps
femoris

40 Posterior Approach to the Knee Joint (Left)

Fig. 40.1 The sigmoid incision runs transversely at the level of the joint line with medial distal and lateral proximal extensions as shown.

Points to consider

- A wider exposure can be obtained by dividing geniculate branches of the popliteal artery.

Position

The patient is prone with the hip and knee extended and a tourniquet around the thigh.

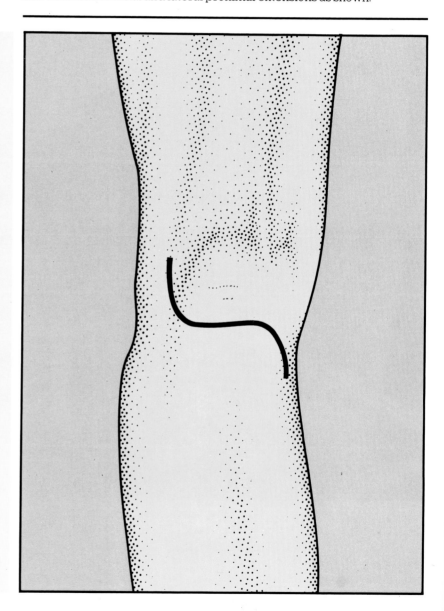

Fig. 40.2 The superficial veins are tied and deep fascia incised.

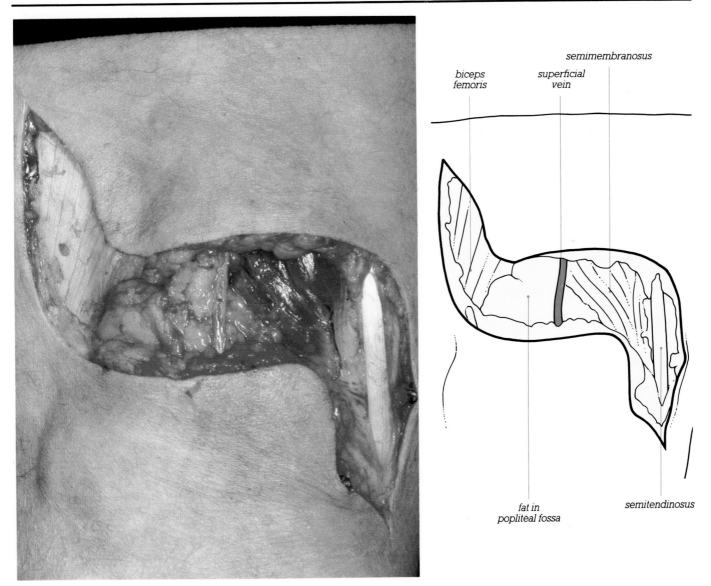

Fig. 40.3 The common peroneal and tibial nerves and the popliteal vein and artery are identified within the fat in the popliteal fossa.

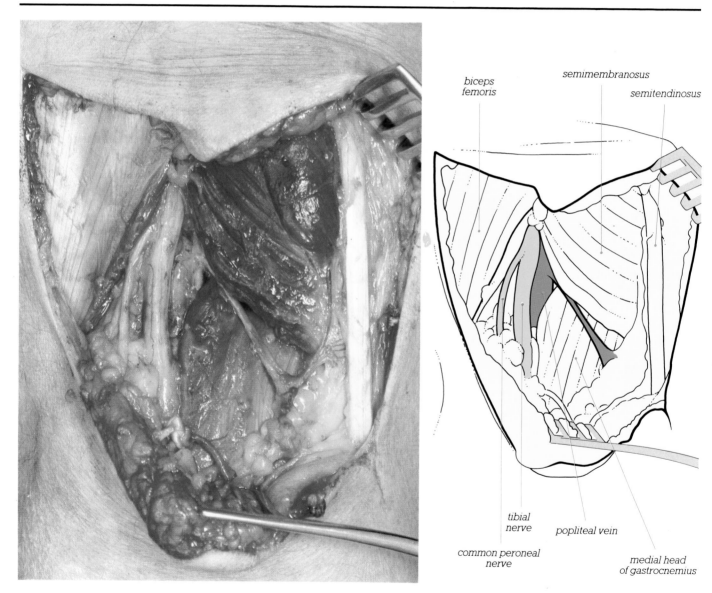

biceps
femoris

semimembranosus

semitendinosus

tibial
nerve

popliteal vein

common peroneal
nerve

medial head
of gastrocnemius

Fig. 40.4 The medial head of gastrocnemius is divided close to its origin on the femur and retracted distally. The middle geniculate artery, which leaves the popliteal artery medially to enter the knee joint, is identified, tied and divided.

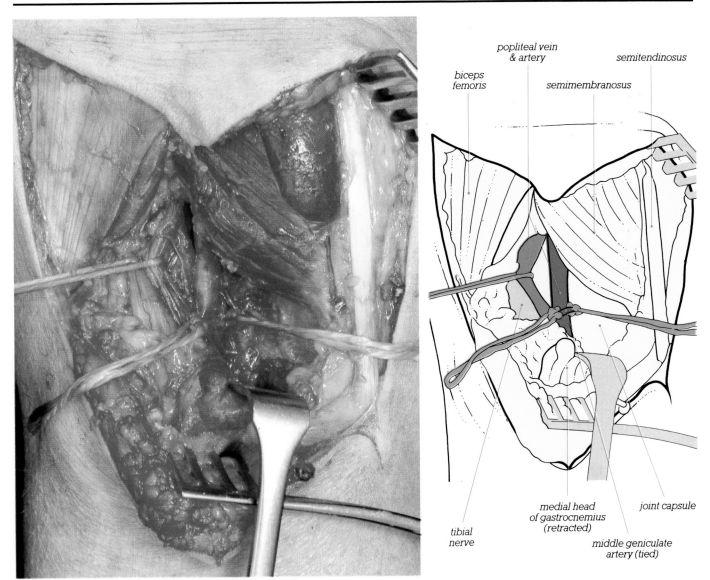

biceps femoris

popliteal vein & artery

semimembranosus

semitendinosus

tibial nerve

medial head of gastrocnemius (retracted)

middle geniculate artery (tied)

joint capsule

2.77

Fig. 40.5 The oblique popliteal ligament, a condensation of the joint capsule, is incised longitudinally.

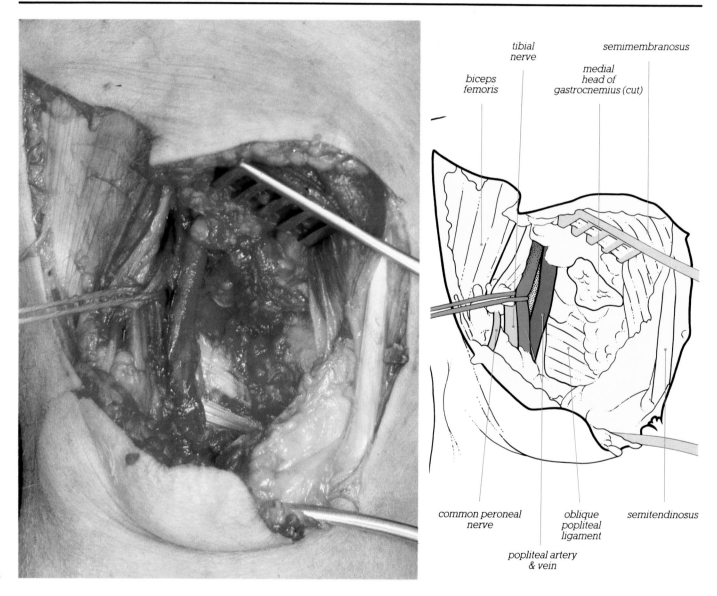

Fig. 40.6 The posterior cruciate ligament can now be identified.

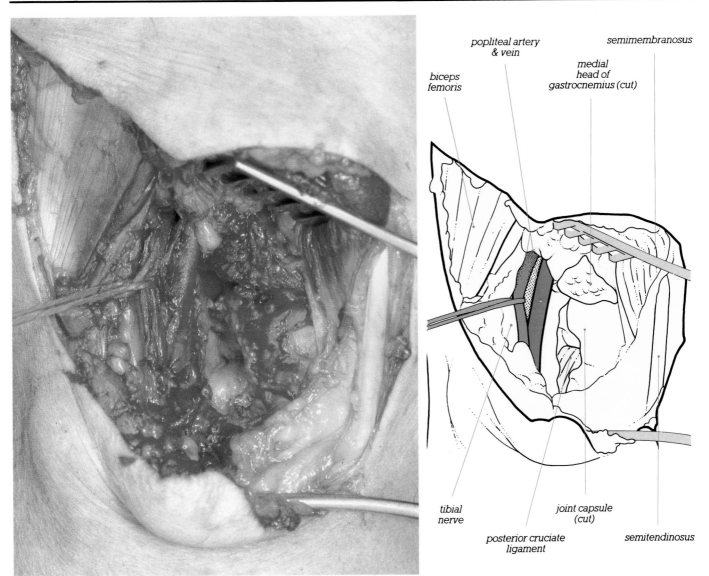

popliteal artery & vein

semimembranosus

biceps femoris

medial head of gastrocnemius (cut)

tibial nerve

joint capsule (cut)

posterior cruciate ligament

semitendinosus

41 Medial Approach to the Distal Popliteal Artery (Left)

Fig. 41.1 The slightly curved incision commences just proximal to the joint line and extends distally parallel to and 1cm behind the medial border of the tibia. It may be extended distally as required (see Figs. 42.1-42.5).

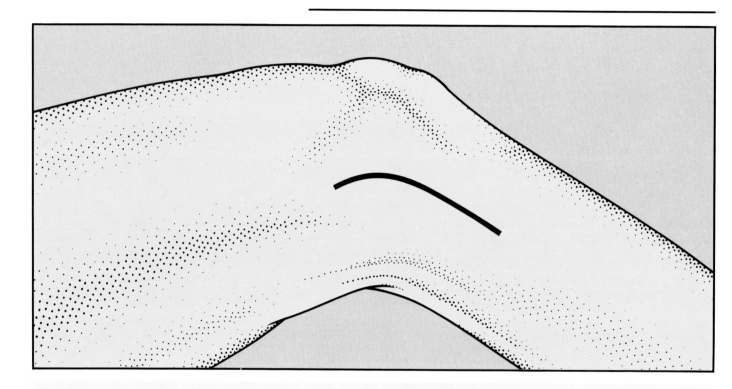

Points to consider

- This exposure is usually used when performing a femoropopliteal bypass.

- If access is limited, exposure is improved if the tendons of sartorius and gracilis are divided. The tendons are repaired at the end of the operation.

Position

The patient is supine with the hip slightly flexed and externally rotated, the knee flexed and supported on a sandbag. No tourniquet is applied.

Fig. 41.2 Taking care to preserve the long saphenous vein if encountered, the superficial and deep fascia are incised in the line of the skin incision. Sartorius is identified proximally and the medial head of gastrocnemius distally.

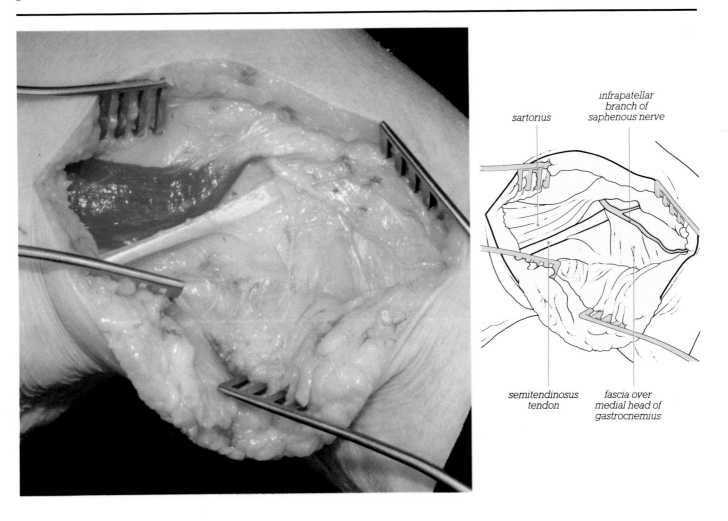

sartorius

infrapatellar branch of saphenous nerve

semitendinosus tendon

fascia over medial head of gastrocnemius

Fig. 41.3 Sartorius and the semitendinosus tendon are retracted upwards and gastrocnemius downwards to expose the fat in the popliteal fossa, which is dissected to expose the popliteal neurovascular structures.

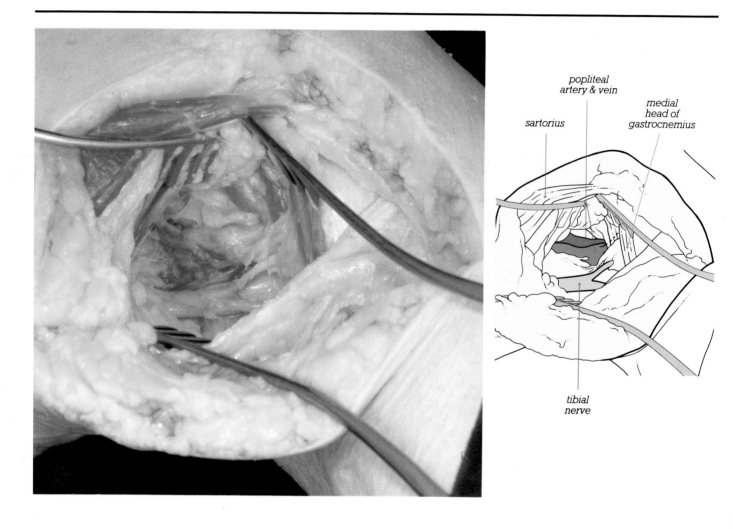

Fig. 41.4 Dissection is carried to the wall of the popliteal artery to free it from the popliteal vein and tibial nerve. Slings placed round the artery proximally and distally are used to retract the artery while identifying branches around which slings are also placed.

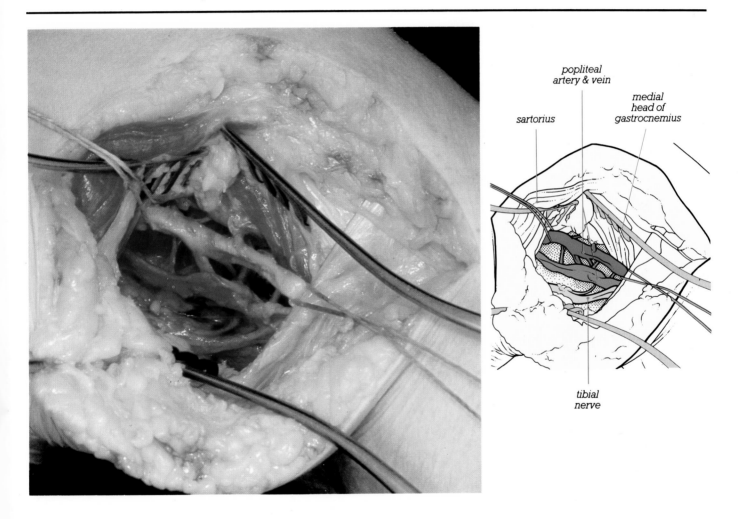

popliteal
artery & vein

medial
head of
gastrocnemius

sartorius

tibial
nerve

42 Exposure of the Bifurcation of the Popliteal Artery (Right)

Fig. 42.1 The incision is longitudinal, parallel to and 1cm behind the upper third of the medial border of the tibia.

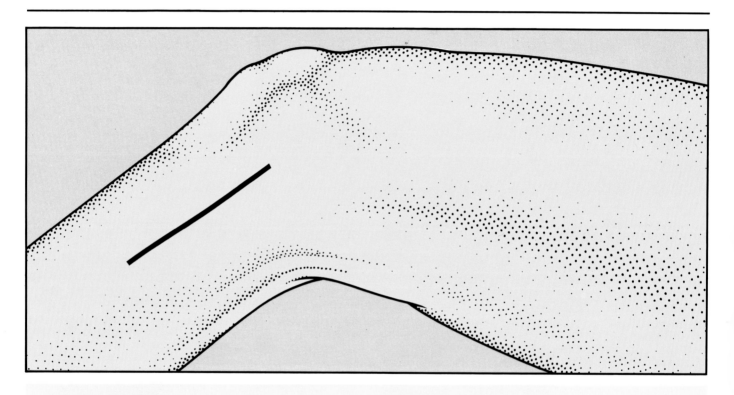

Points to consider

- This exposure is used for a distal femoropopliteal bypass or, when the popliteal artery is completely occluded, a femorotibial bypass.

Position
The patient is supine with the hip slightly flexed and externally rotated, the knee flexed and supported on a sandbag. No tourniquet is applied.

Fig. 42.2 Taking care to preserve the long saphenous vein if encountered, the superficial and deep fascia are incised in the line of the skin incision. The medial head of gastrocnemius is identified inferiorly and the insertions of sartorius, gracilis and semitendinosus into the tibia anteriorly.

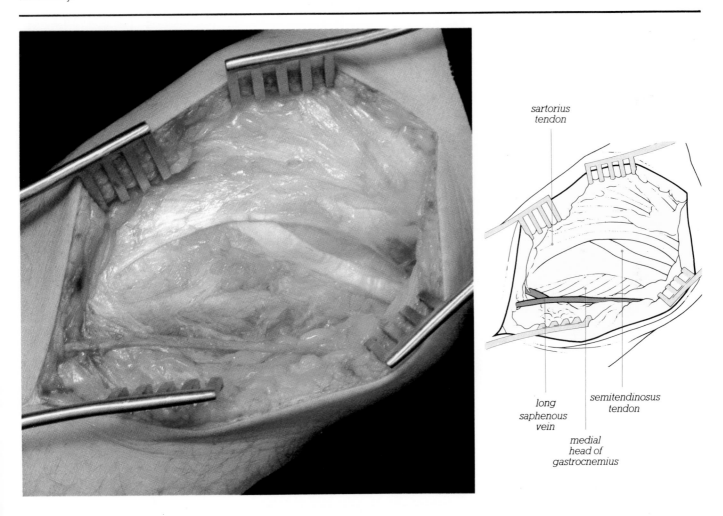

sartorius
tendon

long
saphenous
vein

semitendinosus
tendon

medial
head of
gastrocnemius

Fig. 42.3 Gastrocnemius is retracted inferiorly to expose soleus, and the fibrous attachment of soleus to the tibia and soleal line is divided. After retraction of soleus inferiorly, the distal popliteal artery and vein with the posterior tibial nerve are seen.

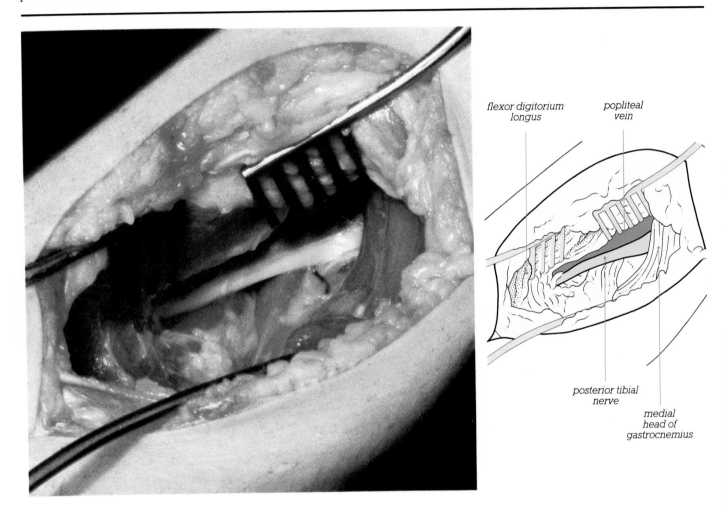

flexor digitorium longus

popliteal vein

posterior tibial nerve

medial head of gastrocnemius

Fig. 42.4 Dissection close to the arterial wall frees the popliteal artery from the vein and nerve.

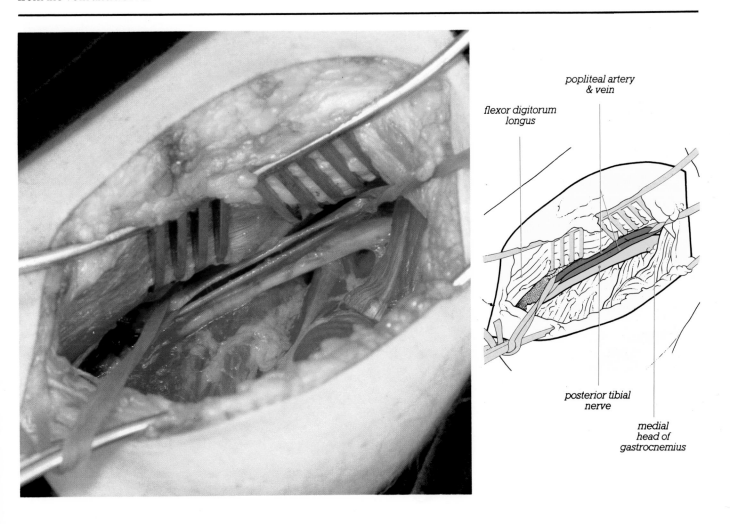

flexor digitorum longus

popliteal artery & vein

posterior tibial nerve

medial head of gastrocnemius

Fig. 42.5 Continuation of the dissection distally along the popliteal artery exposes its bifurcation into anterior and posterior tibial arteries. Slings are placed around the arteries.

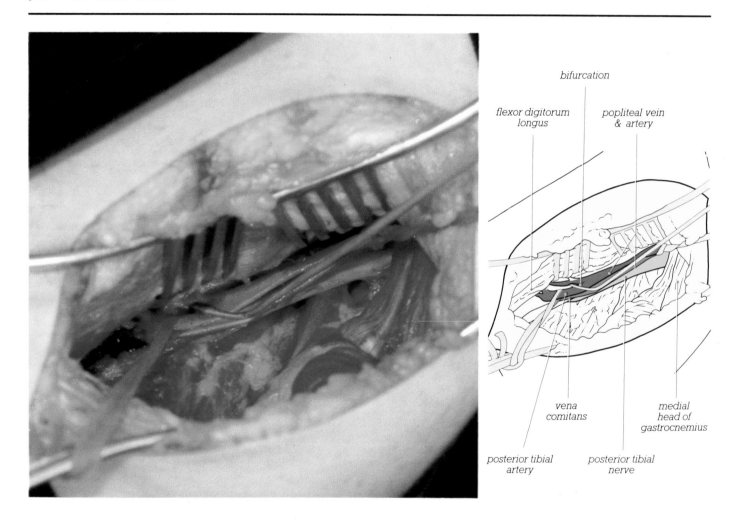

43 Posterolateral Approach to the Tibia and Fibula (Right)

Fig. 43.1 The incision runs along the skin depression behind the fibula.

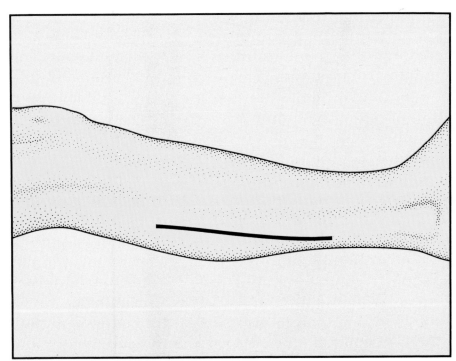

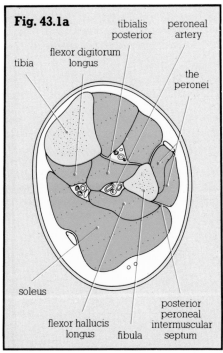

Fig. 43.1a

tibia

flexor digitorum longus

tibialis posterior

peroneal artery

the peronei

soleus

flexor hallucis longus

fibula

posterior peroneal intermuscular septum

Points to consider

- The common peroneal nerve wraps itself around the neck of the fibula and care should be taken not to damage it.

- This posterolateral approach to the tibia is difficult and alternative approaches should first be considered.

Position

The patient is prone or in the lateral position. The affected leg is extended and a tourniquet placed around the thigh.

Fig. 43.2   The incision is continued to the deep fascia and the poorly developed posterior peroneal intermuscular septum identified. The peronei are separated from flexor hallucis longus and soleus by splitting along the posterior peroneal intermuscular septum. Branches of the peroneal artery winding around the fibula are encountered, and are divided as necessary.

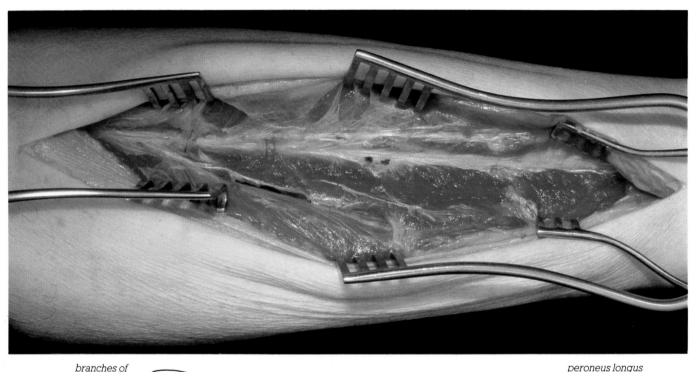

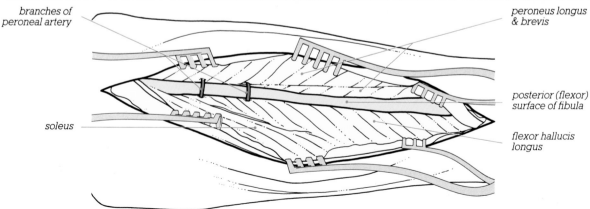

branches of
peroneal artery

soleus

peroneus longus
& brevis

posterior (flexor)
surface of fibula

flexor hallucis
longus

Fig. 43.3 By stripping off flexor hallucis longus, the flexor surface of the fibula is now exposed. The peroneal artery is swept back with flexor hallucis longus.

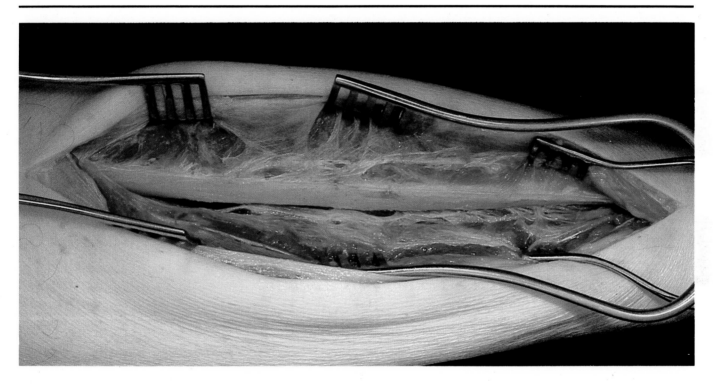

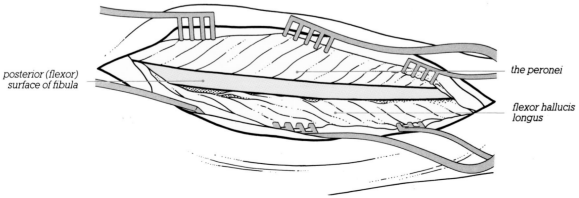

posterior (flexor) surface of fibula

the peronei

flexor hallucis longus

Fig. 43.4 By sweeping tibialis posterior off the interosseous membrane and flexor digitorum longus off the flexor surface of the tibia, the shaft of the tibia is exposed.

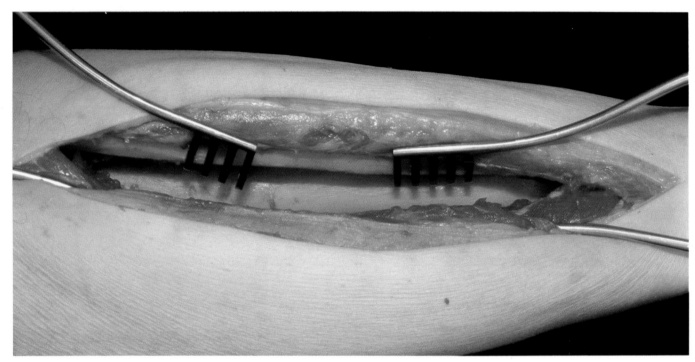

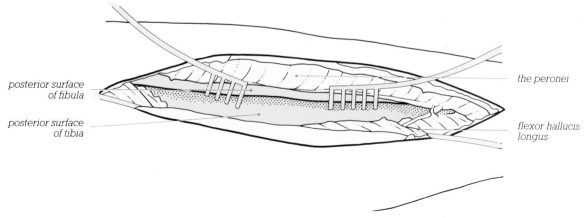

posterior surface of fibula

posterior surface of tibia

the peronei

flexor hallucis longus

44 Anteromedial Approach to the Tibia (Right)

Fig. 44.1 The incision runs longitudinally in the centre of the palpable subcutaneous border of the tibia.

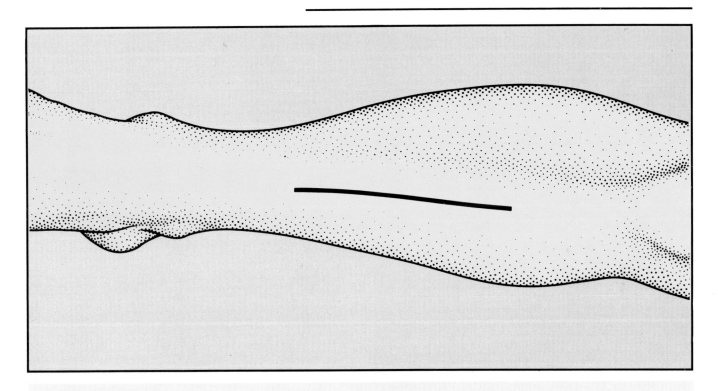

Points to consider

- All lower leg vessels are well protected in this approach.

- Damage to the skin may make this incision unsuitable.

Position

The patient is supine with the hip and knee extended and a tourniquet around the thigh.

Fig. 44.2 The incision is deepened to the periosteum.

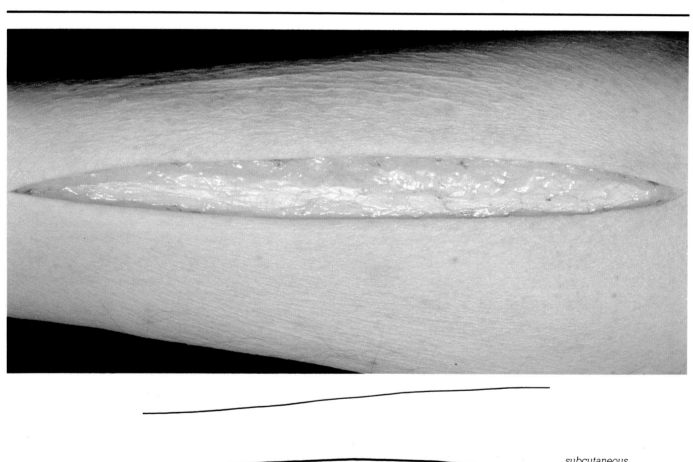

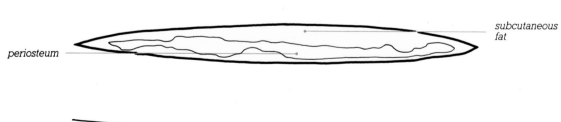

periosteum

subcutaneous
fat

Fig. 44.3 The periosteum is incised and lifted off the tibia.

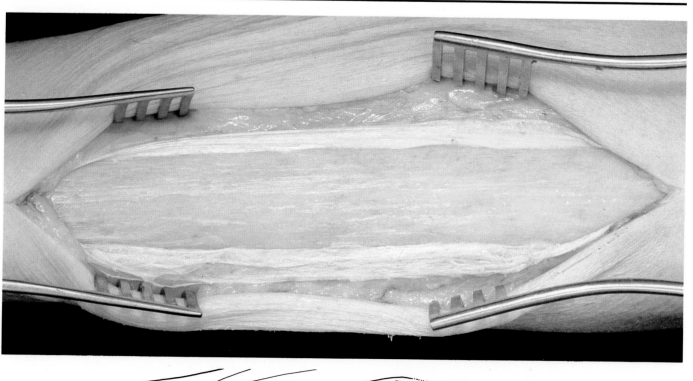

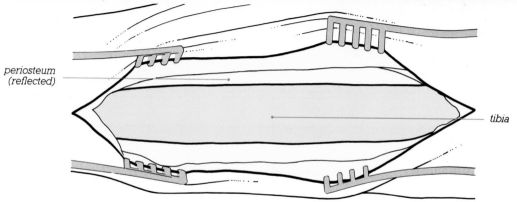

periosteum
(reflected)

tibia

45 Anterolateral Approach to the Tibia (Right)

Fig. 45.1 The incision is 1cm lateral to the anterior crest of the tibia.

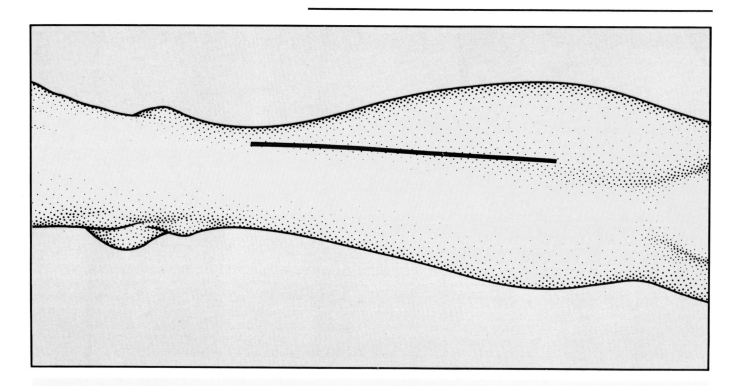

Points to consider

- Damage to the overlying skin may make this incision unsuitable.

Position
The patient is supine with the knee extended and a tourniquet around the thigh.

Fig. 45.2 The incision is deepened to the deep fascia.

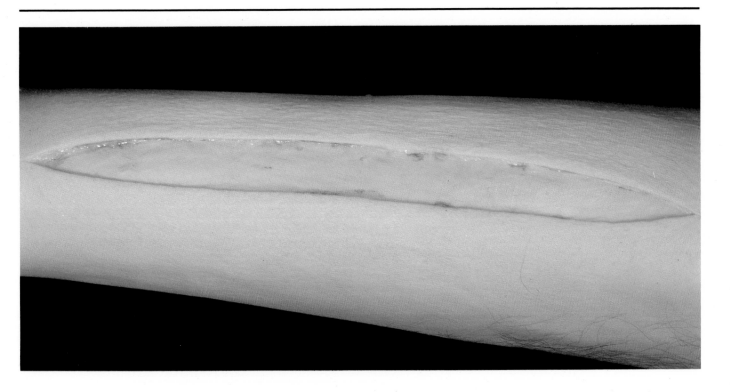

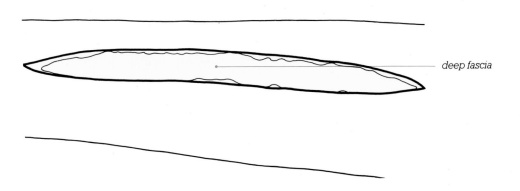

deep fascia

Fig. 45.3 Incision of the deep fascia allows exposure of the anterior muscles of the leg.

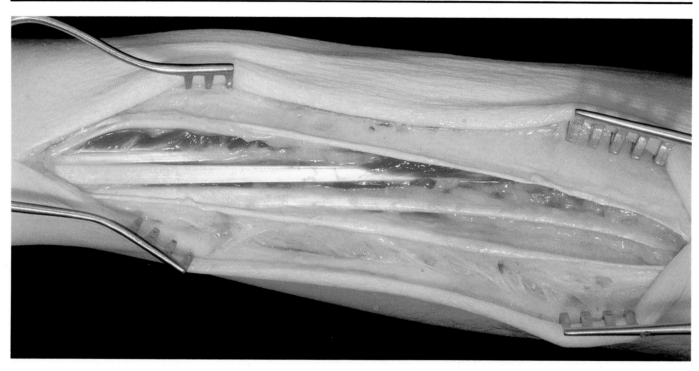

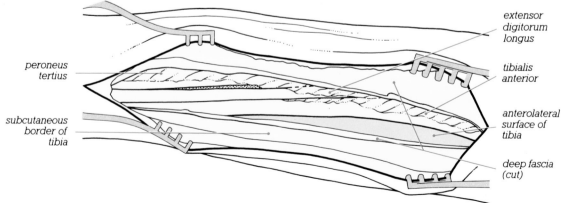

peroneus tertius

subcutaneous border of tibia

extensor digitorum longus

tibialis anterior

anterolateral surface of tibia

deep fascia (cut)

Fig. 45.4 Lateral retraction of tibialis anterior exposes the anterolateral surface of the tibia.

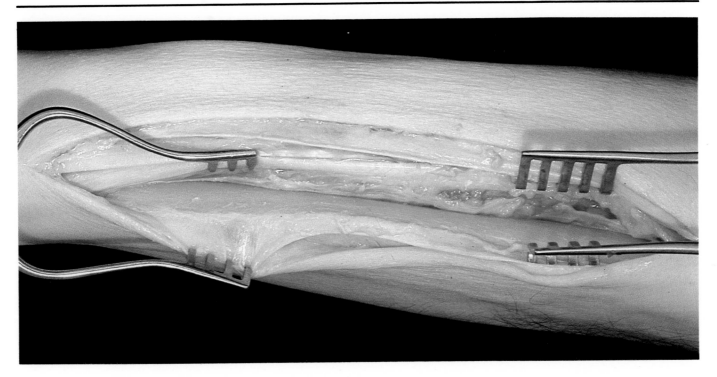

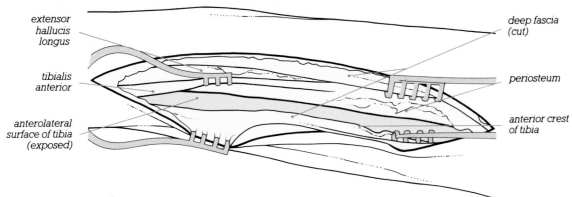

extensor
hallucis
longus

tibialis
anterior

anterolateral
surface of tibia
(exposed)

deep fascia
(cut)

periosteum

anterior crest
of tibia

2.99

46 Posteromedial Approach to the Tibia (Left)

Fig. 46.1 A longitudinal incision is made on the posteromedial aspect of the calf just medial to the line of the tendo Achillis and ends inferiorly at the level of the medial malleolus.

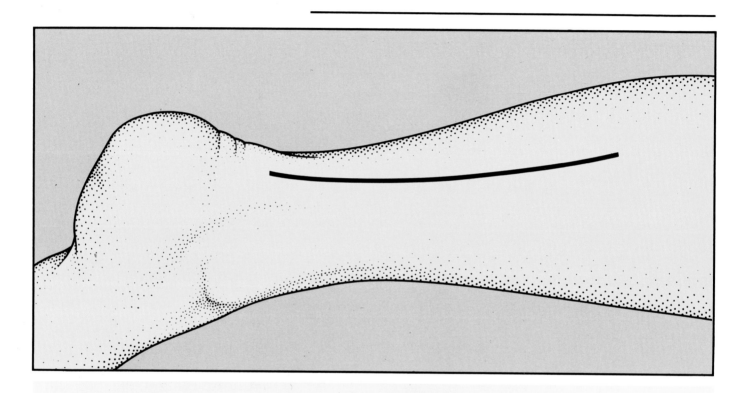

Points to consider

- This approach is useful if there is damage to the skin on the anterior aspect of the lower leg.

- The posterior tibial neurovascular structures are at risk unless they are identified and protected.

Position

The patient is prone with a tourniquet around the thigh. A sandbag under the foot allows slight flexion of the knee.

Fig. 46.2 Dissect through fat to define the tendo Achillis, then carefully dissect deep to the tendon where the posterior tibial neurovascular bundle can be identified, running in the cleft between flexor hallucis longus and flexor digitorum longus.

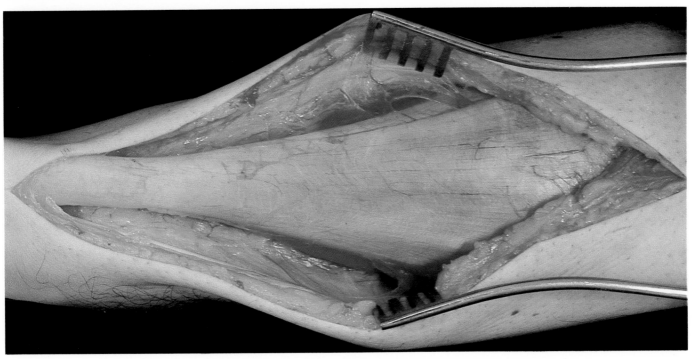

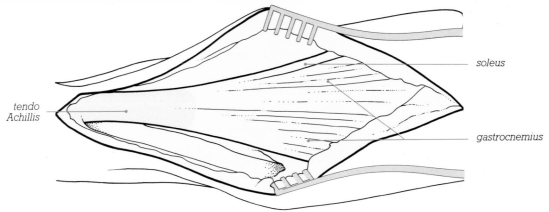

soleus

tendo Achillis

gastrocnemius

Fig. 46.3 After protecting the nerve and vessels with a retractor, a plane opened between the two long flexors exposes the lower third of the tibia. A periosteal elevator is then used to lift the attachments of flexor digitorum longus and tibialis posterior from the tibia to expose the middle third of the tibia.

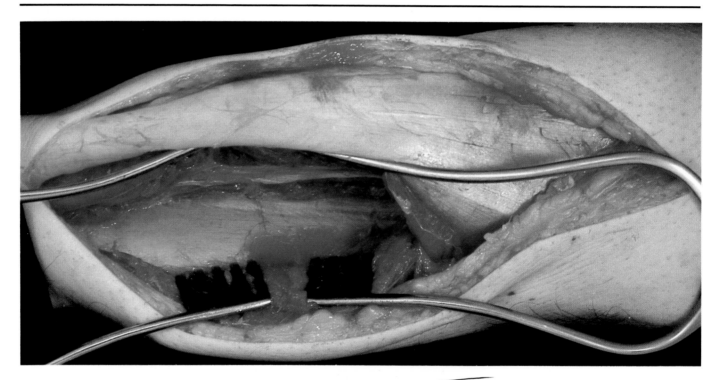

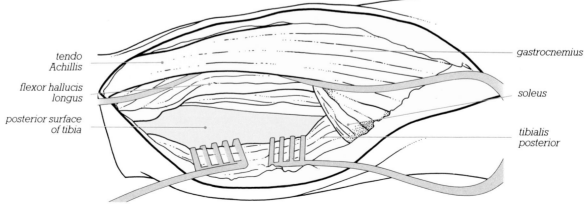

tendo Achillis

flexor hallucis longus

posterior surface of tibia

gastrocnemius

soleus

tibialis posterior

Medial Approach to the Perforating Veins of the Calf (Right)

Fig. 47.1 The incision runs one finger's breadth behind the posterior border of the tibia, from just above the midpoint of the tibia to a point midway between the medial malleolus and the tendo Achillis.

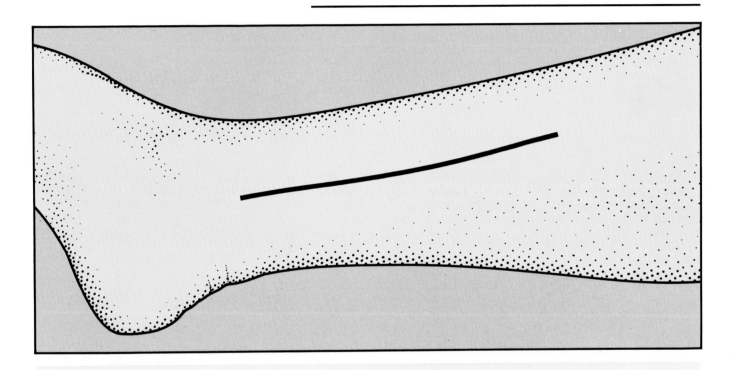

Points to consider

- There are usually three perforators, one posterior to the medial malleolus, one which is four fingers breadth above the medial malleolus and one at about the midpoint of the tibia.

- Sweeping the anterior skin flap off the deep fascia will reveal the long saphenous vein.

- Elevating a skin flap anteriorly or posteriorly before reaching the deep fascia can result in skin necrosis.

- If tissue planes are difficult to find, the deep fascia itself can be raised posteriorly.

Position
The patient is supine, tilted head downwards, and the legs abducted on a vein board.

Fig. 47.2 The incision is deepened down to the deep fascia and the posterior skin swept off to reveal the perforating veins, two of which are demonstrated.

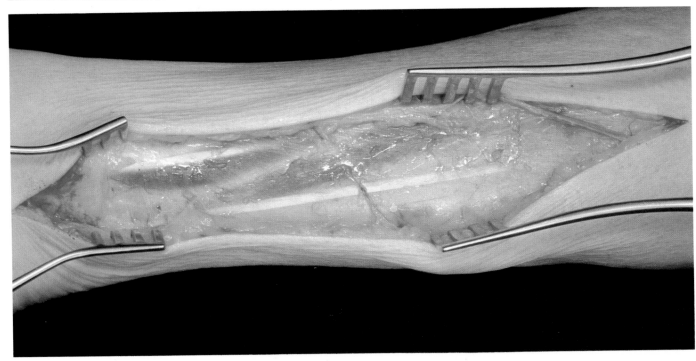

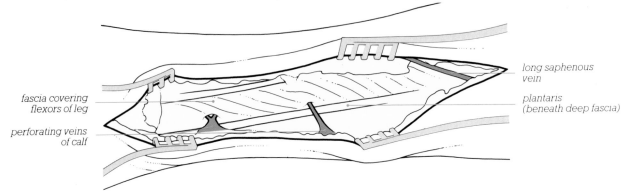

long saphenous vein

plantaris (beneath deep fascia)

fascia covering flexors of leg

perforating veins of calf

Fig. 48.1 The incision runs proximally from the ankle and lies lateral and parallel to the anterior subcutaneous border of the tibia.

Points to consider

- This approach is occasionally used for embolectomy but more frequently is used in distal bypass surgery using the saphenous vein.

Position
The patient is supine with the heel supported and the foot in plantar flexion.

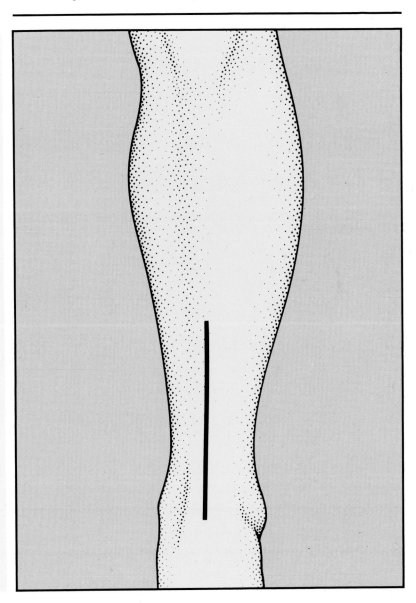

Fig. 48.2 The deep fascia is incised longitudinally in line with the skin incision.

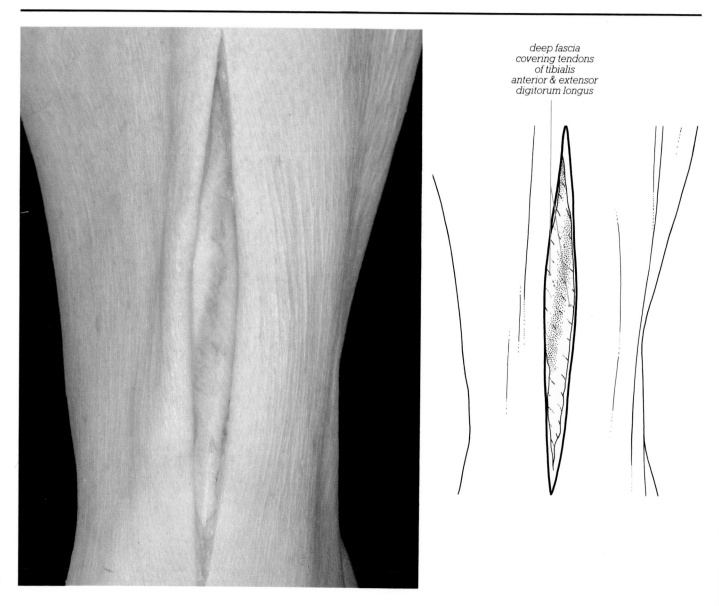

deep fascia
covering tendons
of tibialis
anterior & extensor
digitorum longus

Fig. 48.3 The tendons of tibialis anterior and extensor digitorum longus
are identified and separated. The distal part of extensor hallucis longus is
revealed and may be retracted laterally.

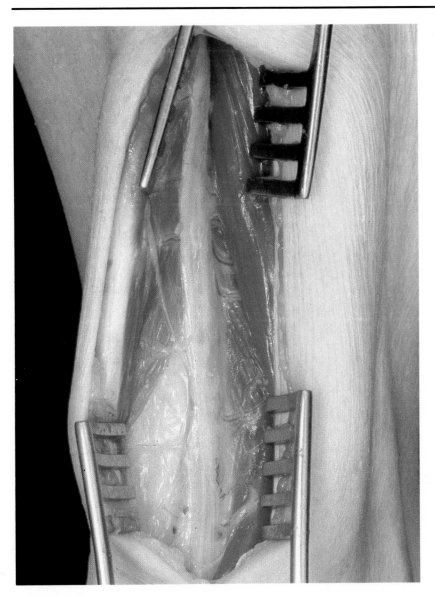

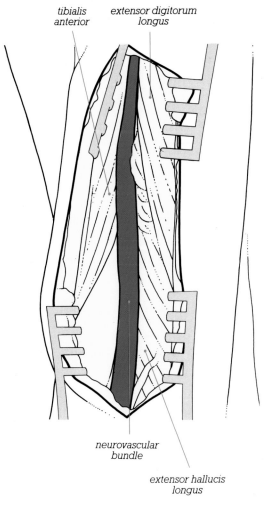

tibialis
anterior

extensor digitorum
longus

neurovascular
bundle

extensor hallucis
longus

2.107

Fig. 48.4 The anterior tibial neurovascular bundle can now be seen lying adjacent to the tibia. After careful dissection of the artery from the nerve and venae comitantes, keeping adjacent to the arterial wall throughout, slings can be passed around the artery proximally and distally.

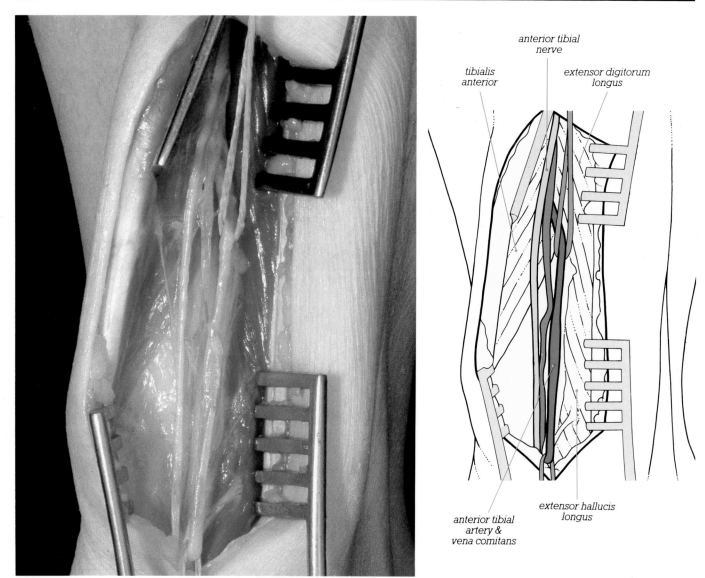

anterior tibial nerve

tibialis anterior

extensor digitorum longus

extensor hallucis longus

anterior tibial artery & vena comitans

49 Anterior Approach to the Ankle Joint (Right)

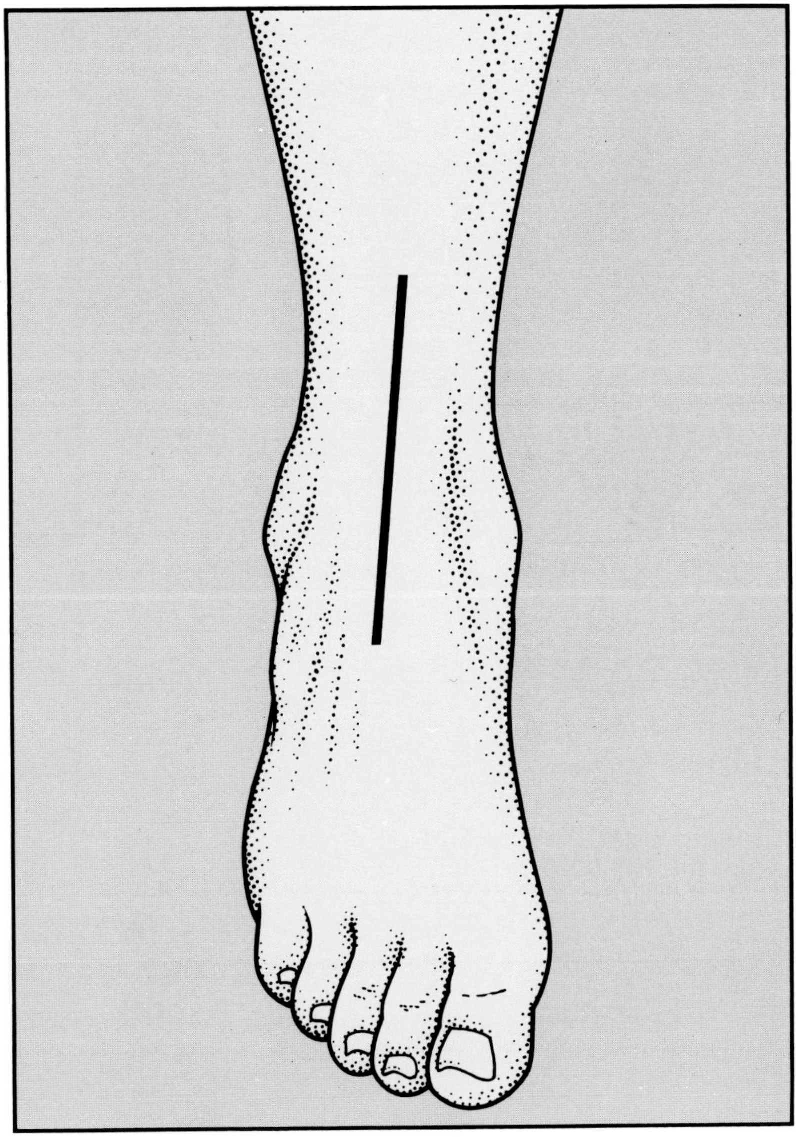

Points to consider

- The superficial peroneal nerve, innervating the dorsum of the foot, lies superficial to the extensor retinacula and should be preserved if seen.

- The deep peroneal nerve runs with the anterior tibial artery and thus is more easily avoided.

Position

The patient is supine with the leg extended and a tourniquet around the thigh.

Fig. 49.1 The vertical incision runs between the tendons of extensor hallucis longus and extensor digitorum longus from 8cm above to 4cm below the joint line.

2.109

Fig. 49.2 The superior and inferior extensor retinacula are incised.

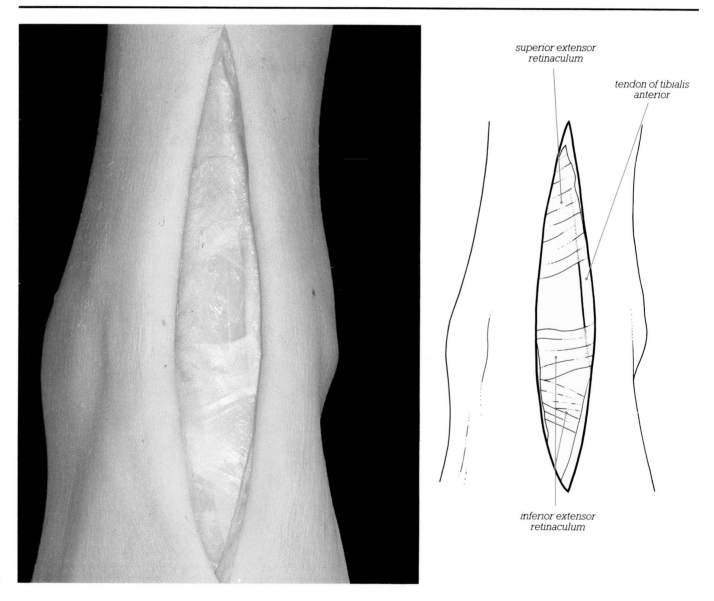

superior extensor
retinaculum

tendon of tibialis
anterior

inferior extensor
retinaculum

Fig. 49.3 Extensor hallucis longus and the anterior tibial artery are retracted medially and extensor digitorum longus retracted laterally to expose the joint capsule.

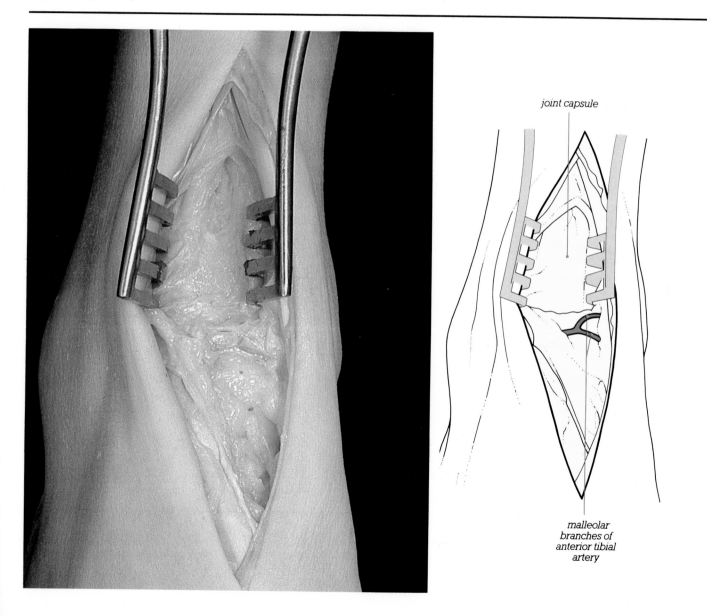

joint capsule

malleolar
branches of
anterior tibial
artery

Fig. 49.4 Incision of the joint capsule opens the ankle joint.

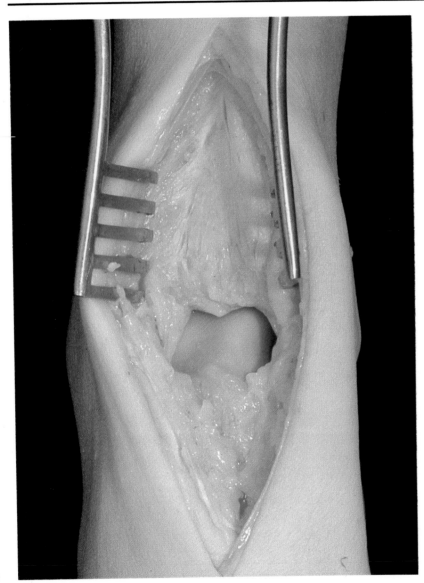

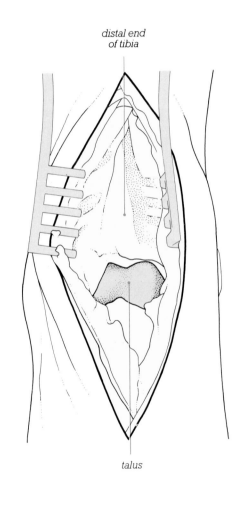

distal end of tibia

talus

50 Exposure of the Medial Malleolus (Left)

Fig. 50.1 The J-shaped incision runs behind and below the malleolus as shown.

Points to consider

- This approach is most frequently used for open reduction and fixation of a fractured malleolus. In these instances the periosteum should be sparingly elevated, particularly on the distal fragment, to reveal just sufficient bone for accurate reduction of the fracture.

- Do not extend the dissection posteriorly as there is a risk of damage to the tendons of tibialis posterior and flexor digitorum longus (see Fig. 50.4), especially when the anatomy is obscured by fracture haematoma.

Position

The patient is supine with the heel supported on a sandbag, the leg externally rotated and a tourniquet around the thigh.

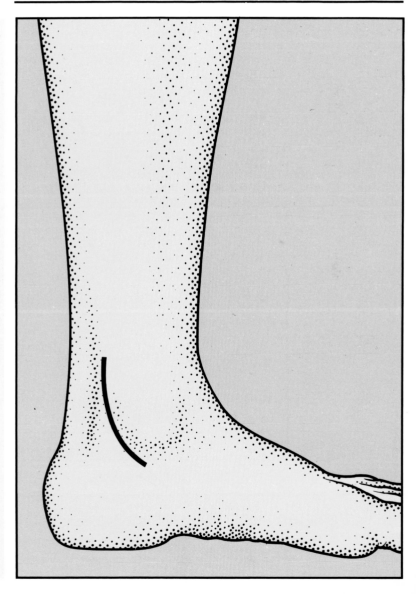

Fig. 50.2 The skin and subcutaneous tissue overlying the malleolus are reflected to fully expose the latter.

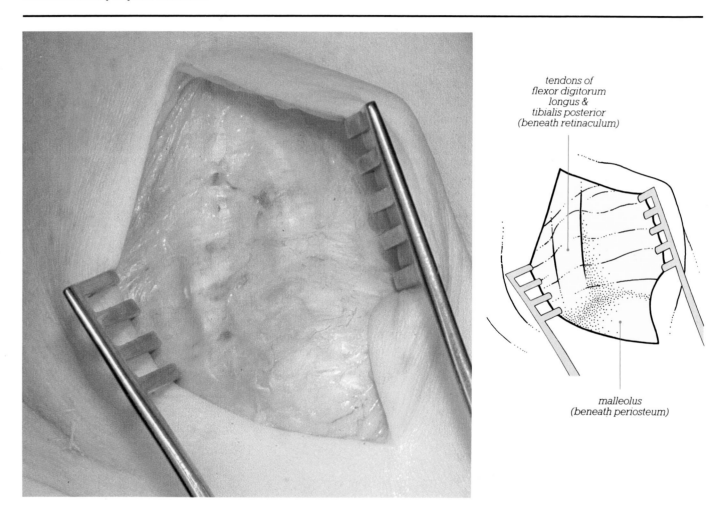

tendons of
flexor digitorum
longus &
tibialis posterior
(beneath retinaculum)

malleolus
(beneath periosteum)

Fig. 50.3 The incision is deepened to the level of the periosteum.
The periosteum is incised and elevated cleanly to expose the bone.

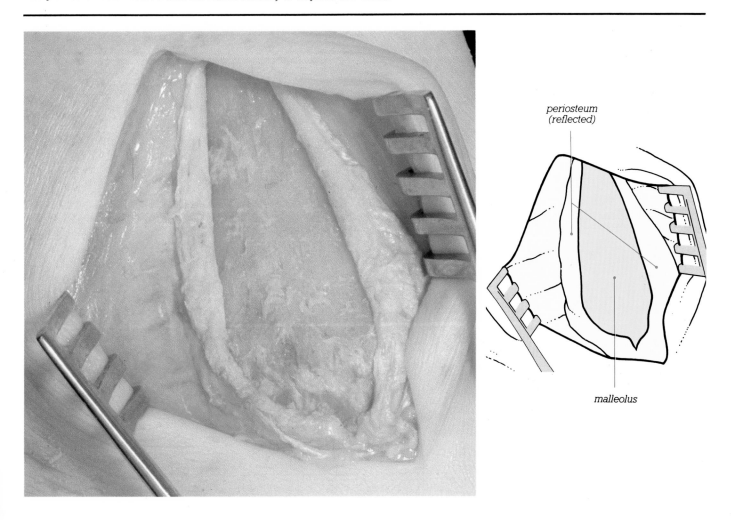

periosteum
(reflected)

malleolus

Fig. 50.4 Extended dissection illustrating the position of the tendons posterior to the malleolus.

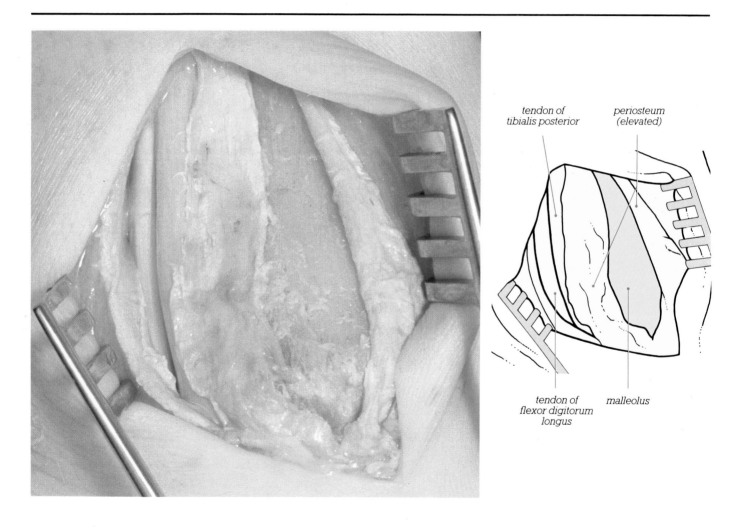

tendon of tibialis posterior

periosteum (elevated)

tendon of flexor digitorum longus

malleolus

1 Exposure of the Lateral Malleolus (Left)

Fig. 51.1 The J-shaped incision runs behind and below the malleolus as shown.

Points to consider

- This approach is most frequently used for open reduction and fixation of a fractured malleolus. In these instances, the periosteum should be sparingly elevated, particularly on the distal fragment, to reveal just sufficient bone for accurate reduction of the fracture.

- Do not extend the dissection too far posteriorly as there is a risk of damage to the tendons of peroneus longus and brevis (see Fig. 51.3), especially when the anatomy is obscured by fracture haematoma.

Position

The patient is supine with the heel supported on a sandbag, a large sandbag under the ipsilateral buttock to ensure internal rotation of the leg and a tourniquet around the thigh.

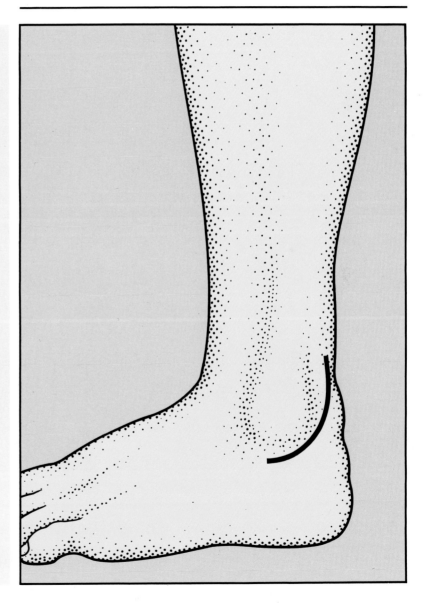

Fig. 51.2 The incision is deepened onto the periosteum and the skin and subcutaneous tissue reflected anteriorly to expose the tendons posterior to the malleolus. The periosteum is incised and elevated to expose the bone.

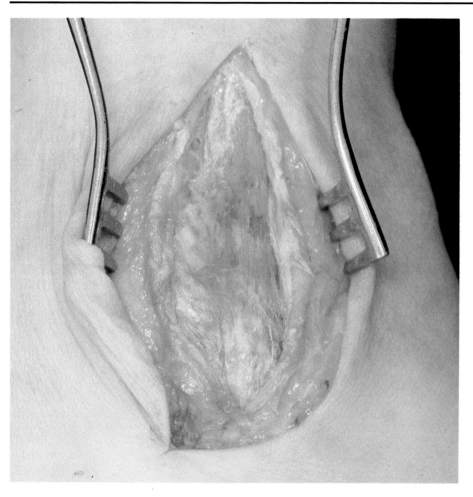

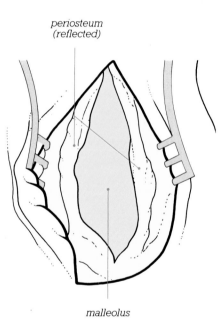

periosteum
(reflected)

malleolus

Fig. 51.3 Extended dissection illustrating the position of the tendons posterior to the malleolus.

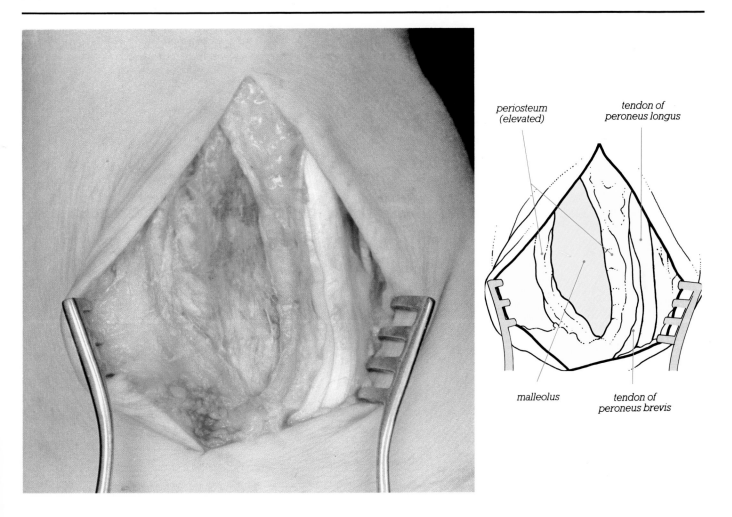

periosteum
(elevated)

tendon of
peroneus longus

malleolus

tendon of
peroneus brevis

52 Exposure of the Tendo Achillis (Right)

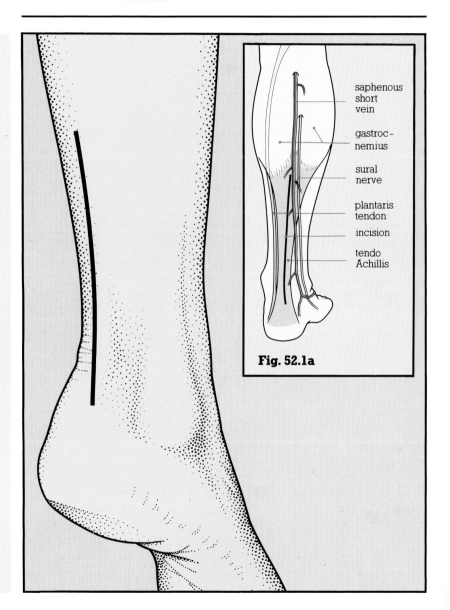

Fig. 52.1 The longitudinal incision runs down the midline of the calf, bearing slightly laterally in the lower part of the incision to avoid making a scar over the calcaneum.

Points to consider

- This approach is usually used to repair a ruptured tendo Achillis. If rupture is complete it may be necessary to extend the incision proximally for adequate access to the proximal stump of the tendon. In this case a preserved plantaris tendon can be used to repair the rupture.

Fig. 52.1a

saphenous
short
vein

gastroc-
nemius

sural
nerve

plantaris
tendon

incision

tendo
Achillis

Position

The patient is prone with a tourniquet around the thigh. The leg is supported by a sandbag beneath the foot.

2.120

Fig. 52.2 Taking care to preserve the sural nerve and short saphenous vein, the dissection is deepened as far as the paratenon on the tendo Achillis. If a plantaris tendon is found on the medial side of the tendo Achillis, preserve it (see Fig. 52.1a). The tendo Achillis can be fully demonstrated by dissecting away the fatty tissue lying between it and the long flexors to the foot and the posterior tibial neurovascular bundle.

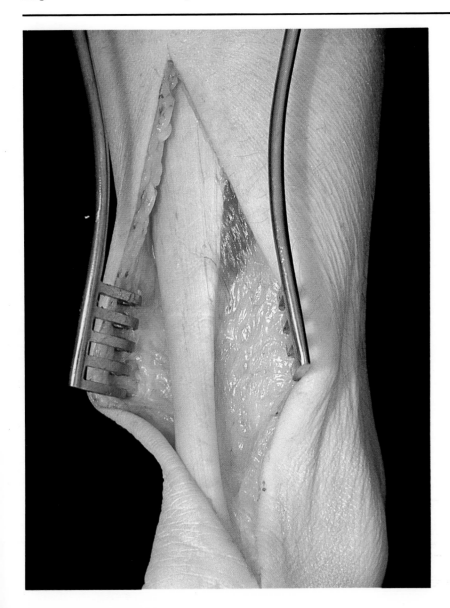

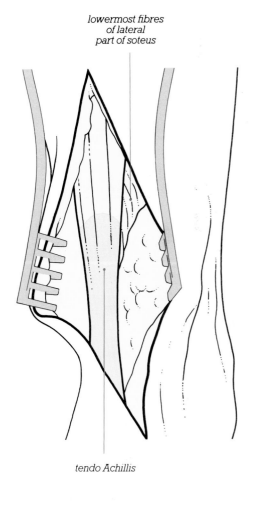

lowermost fibres
of lateral
part of soteus

tendo Achillis

53 Exposure of the Posterior Malleolus (Left)

2.122

Fig. 53.1 The incision begins a thumb's breadth below the lateral malleolus and curves to the lateral border of the tendo Achillis to run about 12cm up the leg.

Points to consider

- More tibia can be exposed by detaching the lowermost attachment of flexor hallucis longus from the fibula.

- The short saphenous vein runs behind the lateral malleolus to the posterior aspect of the calf.

- Branches of the sural nerve, supplying the posterior aspect of the calf and the lateral aspect of the foot, run in the same direction as the skin incision.

Position

The patient is prone with a tourniquet around the thigh. A small sandbag under the dorsum of the foot allows some flexion of the knee and plantar flexion of the foot.

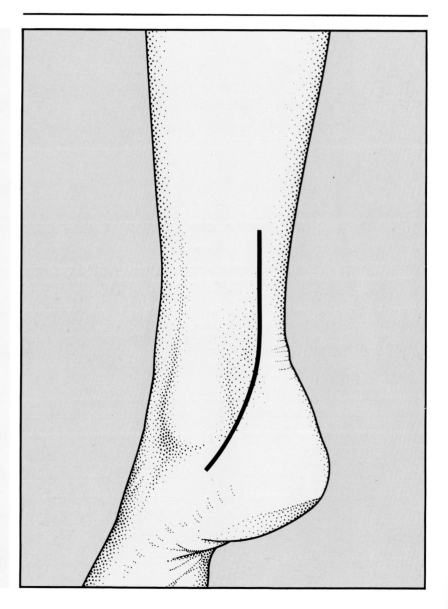

Fig. 53.2 The incision is deepened to expose the tendo Achillis and flexor hallucis longus. Tendo Achillis is elevated, revealing the posterior tibial nerve and peroneal artery.

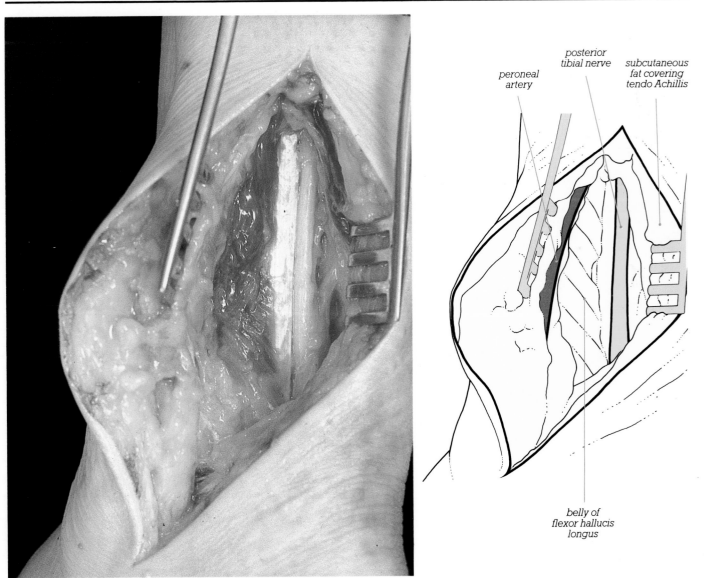

peroneal
artery

posterior
tibial nerve

subcutaneous
fat covering
tendo Achillis

belly of
flexor hallucis
longus

Fig. 53.3 Avoiding damage to the peroneal artery, the interval between flexor hallucis longus and the peroneal muscles is developed. Flexor hallucis longus is retracted medially to reveal the posterior malleolus.

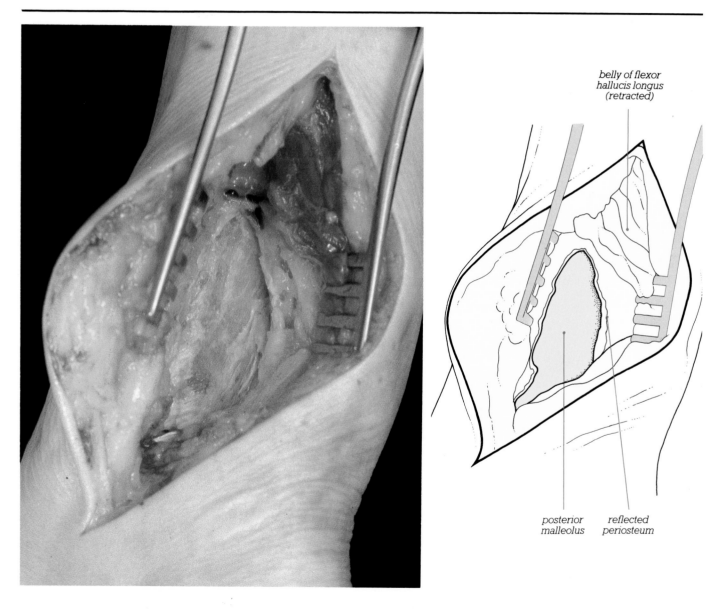

belly of flexor
hallucis longus
(retracted)

posterior
malleolus

reflected
periosteum

Exposure of the Posterior Tibial Artery at the Ankle (Left)

Fig. 54.1 The incision runs vertically behind the medial malleolus.

Points to consider

- This exposure may be used for exploration preparatory to performing a distal bypass procedure and when creating an arteriovenous (for example, Scribner) shunt for use in haemodialysis.

Position

The patient is supine with the leg externally rotated. No tourniquet is used

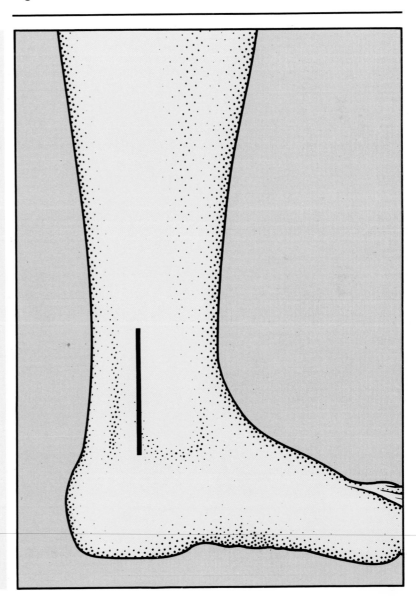

Fig. 54.2 The superficial fascia is incised in the line of the skin incision to reveal the neurovascular bundle just beneath the deep fascia.

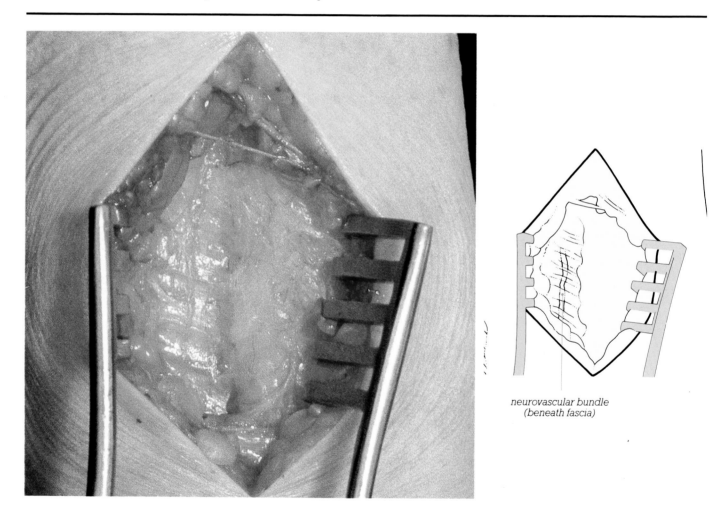

neurovascular bundle
(beneath fascia)

Fig. 54.3 The deep fascia is incised in the line of the neurovascular bundle, and the posterior tibial artery dissected away from its venae comitantes and the posterior tibial nerve. Slings are placed round the artery proximally and distally.

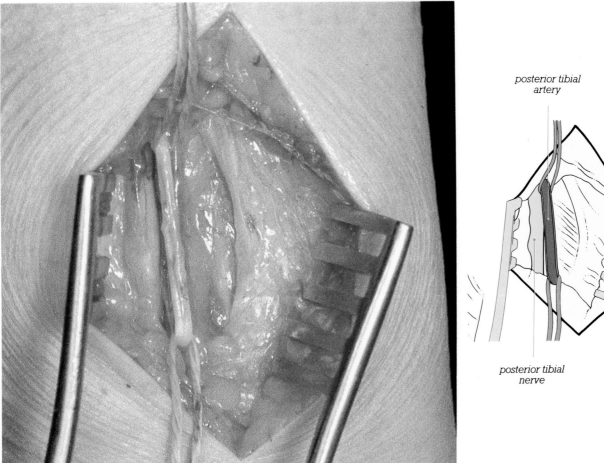

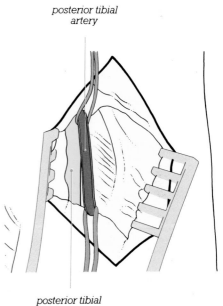

posterior tibial
artery

posterior tibial
nerve

55 Medial Approach to the First Metatarsophalangeal Joint (Left)

Fig. 55.1 The 6cm incision runs along the medial aspect of the first metatarsal across the joint line, then curves to run along the medial aspect of the proximal phalanx to its midpoint.

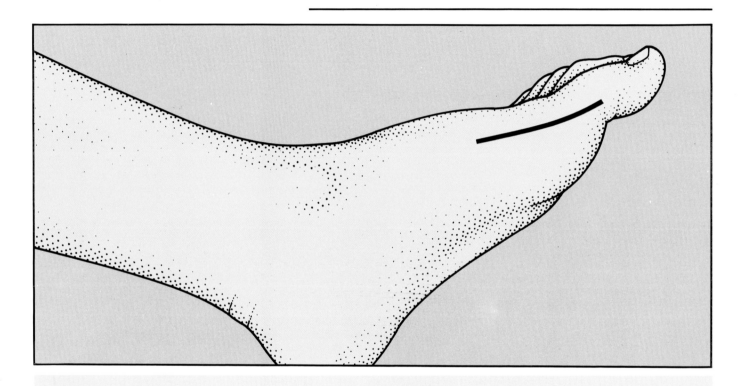

Points to consider

- The incision can be extended proximally or distally.

- The main digital nerve, which supplies the medial side of the hallux, lies plantar to this incision.

Position

The patient is supine with the leg extended and a tourniquet around the thigh.

Fig. 55.2 The incision is deepened, avoiding the terminal branch of the superficial peroneal nerve which supplies the dorsal aspect of the great toe.

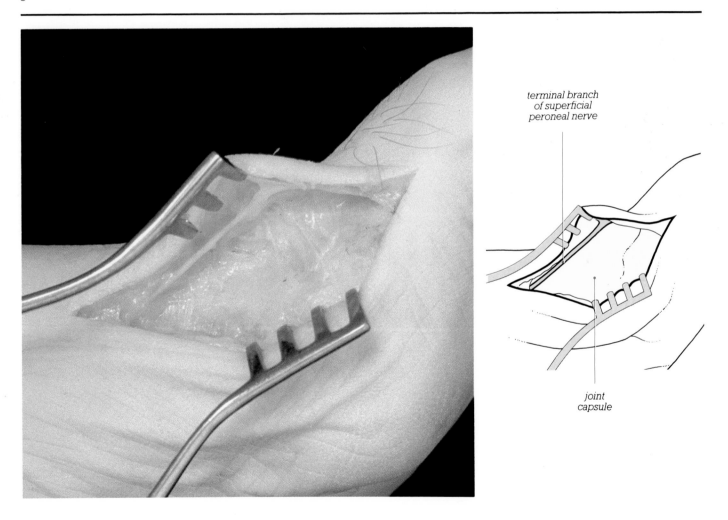

terminal branch
of superficial
peroneal nerve

joint
capsule

Fig. 55.3 The capsule is incised along the same line as the skin incision.

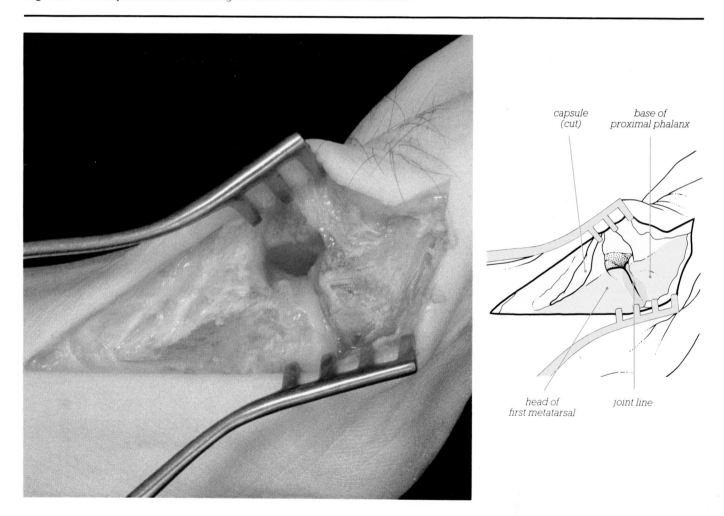

capsule (cut)

base of proximal phalanx

head of first metatarsal

joint line